# ABCs of
# CANCER

# ABCs of CANCER

## Tips for Teens to
## Help a Parent Survive

KATHERINE CARR
AND JACQUELINE CARR

Forewords by
Steven DeMeester, M.D.
and Michael Hu, M.D.

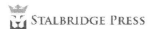 STALBRIDGE PRESS

## MEDICAL DISCLAIMER

This book is based on the personal experiences of the authors and is not intended as a medical manual. The information should not be considered a substitute for the advice of medical, financial or other professionals. The authors do not recommend or endorse any specific tests, physicians, products, procedures, opinions, or other information mentioned in this book. The authors expressly disclaim responsibility for any adverse effects resulting from the application of the information in this book.

All photos by Jacqueline Carr and Katherine Carr except the front and back covers, by Carol Cirillo Stanley, p. xiii courtesy Steven DeMeester, M.D., p. xvii courtesy Michael Hu, M.D. p. xviii courtesy Kids Konnected, p. 22 courtesy Ed Mitchell, p. 29 Darlene Miller, p. 64-192 and small animal silhouettes iStock.com.

ABCs of CANCER: Tips for Teens to Help a Parent Survive
Copyright 2016 Katherine Carr and Jacqueline Carr
www.StalbridgePress.com
stalbridgepress@gmail.com

ISBN: 0996488243
ISBN 13: 9780996488243
Library of Congress Control Number: 2016901223
Stalbridge Press, Irvine CA

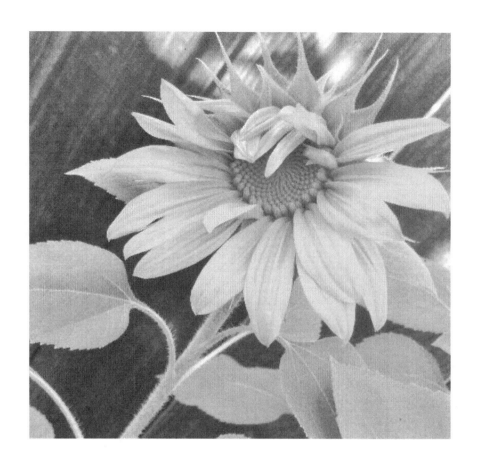

# CONTENTS

# OUR ROADMAP – DIAGNOSIS TO SURGERY PRE-OP

# OUR ROADMAP – SURGERY TO RECOVERY

Jacqueline Carr — Age 14-15 at time of mother's cancer

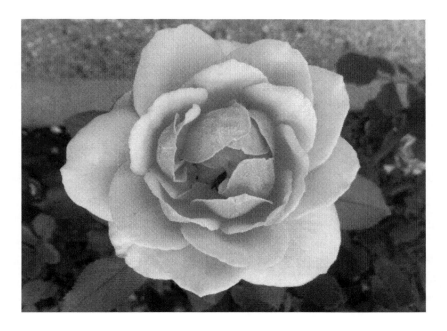

# ABCs of CANCER – 127 TIPS, TERMS & TIDBITS

## A

Alarm, Alkaline, American Cancer Society, Apps   63

## B

Benign, Biopsy, Brighten (The Home), Books   68

## C

Cancer Compass, CaringBridge, Case Manager, Chemo Brain & Chemo Curls, Chemotherapy, Clinical Trials, Cold, College, Complications, CT Scan, Cure Magazine   73

## D

Decorating (The Hospital Room), Deep Vein Thrombosis (DVT), Dentist, Designer Barf Bags, Disability, Disabled Parking Permit, Doctors, Driving   82

## E

Emergency Room (ER), Encouragement, Energy, Esophageal Cancer Symptoms, Exercise   87

## F

Face Mask, Feeding Tube, Fending (For Oneself), Finances, Food, Friends & Family   93

# O

Oncologist, Optimistic, Organic, Organizations   142

# P

Pain, Party!, PET Scan, Pets, Physical Therapy (PT), pH Level, PICC Line,   Post-Op & Pre-Op, Prayer, Protein, PubMed, Pulmonary Embolism (PE)   146

# Q

Questions, Quiet   155

# R

Radiation, Radiation Oncologist,   Recurrence,   Research, Risks, Role Reversal   158

# S

Schedule, School, Side Effects, Sleep, Staging, Statistics, Sugar   163

# T

Teachers, Team, Tears, Tenacity, Treatment, Tumor   168

# U

Ultrasound, Unbelievable   172

# V

Vegan, Vegetables   175

# W

# X

# Y

# Z

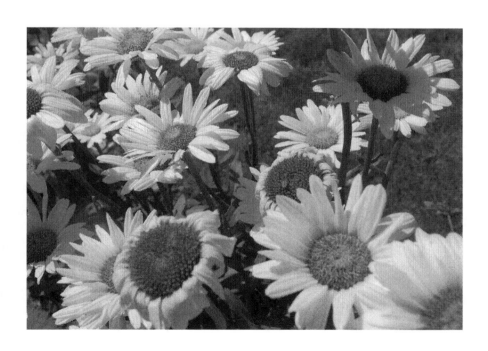

# FOREWORD

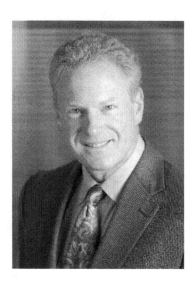

STEVEN DeMEESTER M.D.
Keck Hospital of USC

Cancer. It is a dreaded word, and often associated with huge physical and emotional upheaval in the life of that person and those around them.

Surgeons like myself who daily care for patients with cancer can all too easily allow the empathy for these patients to dissipate, or to forget how devastating a cancer diagnosis is for them and their family.

In the "ABCs of Cancer" Katherine and Jacqueline Carr share their mother's journey with esophageal cancer, the fastest increasing cancer in the United States and one of the world's deadliest cancers.

It is a heartfelt account that restores empathy for those who deal with cancer frequently, and helps alley the fears and uncertainties of what comes next for those new to the disruptive world of cancer.

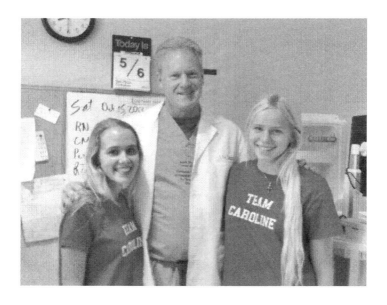

*Dr. DeMeester with Katherine Carr, left and Jacqueline Carr at the ICU a few days after their mother's surgery.*

I clearly remember even several years after their mother Caroline's surgery how involved the girls were as cheerleaders and supporters for their mother during her recovery, and how cohesive the three of them were together, right down to the "Team Caroline" T-shirts that were created. They even gave one to me!

Congratulations to Katherine and Jacqueline for this book and for their incredible dedication to their mother during her treatment and recovery from esophageal cancer. You are both exemplary role models for all children with a parent who has cancer or other life-threatening illness.

*Steven DeMeester, M.D. is a Professor of Surgery at Keck School of Medicine of USC and board certified in General Surgery and Cardiovascular and Thoracic Surgery.*

*As an international leader in the field of esophageal surgery, patients from around the globe travel to be treated by him. He has authored or co-authored over 130 peer-reviewed papers and 15 book chapters, and given invited lectures around the world.*

*In 2013, Dr. DeMeester successfully performed an eight-hour surgery on Katherine and Jacqueline's mother to remove her esophagus to treat her stage 3 esophageal cancer.*

# FOREWORD

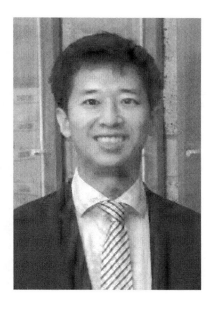

Michael Hu, M.D., M.P.H., M.S.
Stanford University, Kids Konnected

Jon Wagner-Holtz founded Kids Konnected at age 11 after his mother was diagnosed with breast cancer. As a childhood friend of Jon, and now a member of the board of directors at Kids Konnected, I am familiar with the challenges facing teens whose parents have cancer. Our non-profit organization meets the emotional needs of kids by providing support groups and camps where they can interact with others undergoing a similar struggle.

The "ABCs of CANCER" supplies teens with the tools and encouragement for a hands-on approach to a parent with cancer.

It includes everything a teen may want to know, from where to get free wigs for cancer patients to an overview of what to expect when a parent undergoes treatment with chemotherapy, radiation, and/or surgery.

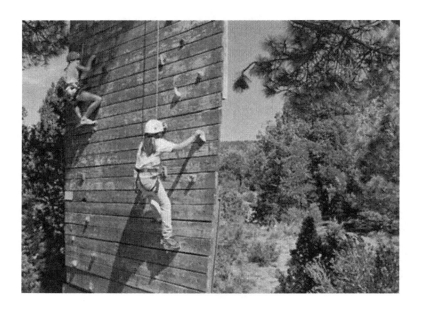

*Teens climbing at a Kids Konnected camp.*

Katherine and Jacqueline helped their mother organize medical information, find a surgeon, and assisted with activities of daily living. In so doing, they helped her increase her odds of survival. The sisters, who were 14 and 17 when their mother was diagnosed, guide us through their journey.

I met Jacqueline about a year and a half after her mother's treatment. Her interest in science and medicine increased after spending time in the hospital caring for her mother.

To pursue this interest, she participated in a research program in stem cell biology at Stanford University, where I am a post-doctoral fellow.

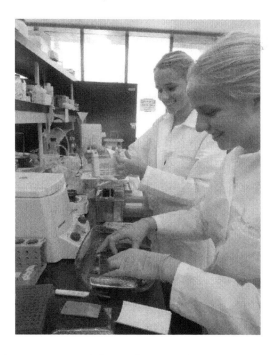

*Katherine Carr, left, and Jacqueline Carr perform cancer research at the University of California, Irvine in 2014.**

Reading the "ABCs of CANCER" will take you through the challenge of having a parent with cancer. Written from two perspectives, it will guide teens through the journey with the help of two friends. With over 50 photos and 120 tips, the book is like no other I have ever read about cancer. I highly recommend it for any teen who is facing this difficult challenge.

*Michael Hu, M.D., M.P.H., M.S. is a general surgery resident training to become a craniofacial plastic surgeon.*

*He is on the board of directors of Kids Konnected, a non-profit organization that supports kids and teens of parents who have cancer or who have died from cancer. Dr. Hu is currently undergoing a post-doctoral research fellowship in the Hagey Laboratory for Pediatric Regenerative Medicine at Stanford University.*

*\* $1 from the sale of each "ABCs of CANCER" will be donated to cancer research at universities.*

# INTRODUCTION

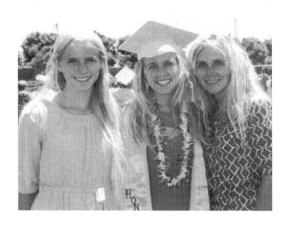

*A week before Katherine graduated from high
school, her mother was diagnosed with cancer.
Jacqueline, left, age 14, Katherine, age 17,
and their mother in June 2013.*

As teens, my daughters Katherine and Jacqueline Carr played a crucial role in enabling me to go from Stage 3 cancer of the esophagus to cancer free in four months.

I followed a traditional medical course for treatment with chemotherapy, radiation and surgery. However, I believe it was my daughters' help in encouraging me through the traditional treatments, and in keeping me focused on following the complementary cancer treatments we had read about in books that helped make the difference to my results. My surgeon described my outcome as phenomenal.

This book details the actions my daughters took to help me. From alkaline water, juicing, organic foods and brightening up our home, to researching the disease, meeting with doctors and helping me during and after surgery, they share their tips from every level of our lives dealing with cancer.

The tables had turned.

Since my daughters were born, they were always the priority in my life and I put their needs first.

Now all of a sudden I came first. I had to come first if we were going to accomplish everything that was needed for me to survive this aggressive cancer — a cancer with a 15 percent five-year survival rate.

I am now two years out from the treatment and have been fortunate so far that there is no sign of a recurrence of the cancer — a cancer with a 70 percent recurrence rate

I am grateful to the excellent doctors I had who successfully treated my cancer with traditional treatments. Dr. Steven DeMeester, Thoracic Surgeon at USC Keck, was a lifesaver. I am amazed by the support of my daughters who continue to encourage me. They grew to be very strong as our family faced cancer.

I am just happy to be alive.

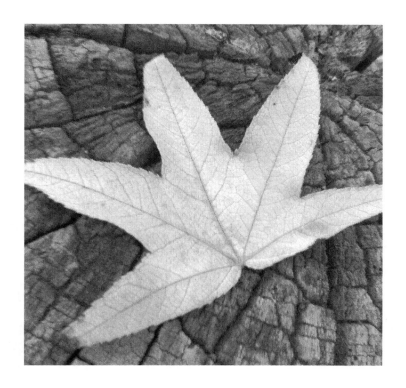

# OUR ROAD MAP –
# DIAGNOSIS TO PRE-OP

By
KATHERINE CARR
*Age 17 at time of mother's cancer*

## GETTING THE NEWS

Here we are, sitting in our living room. Our mom reading on one end of the couch, my sister, Jacqueline, reading on the other. So peaceful. Who would have thought the last six months ever occurred? It seems like a world away now.

Flashback to my last week of high school before I graduated. Everyone was celebrating, laughing and enjoying the end.

But my family was bracing for what was to come.

Cancer—a word everyone hates. A word everyone fears. For some reason I never thought much of it.

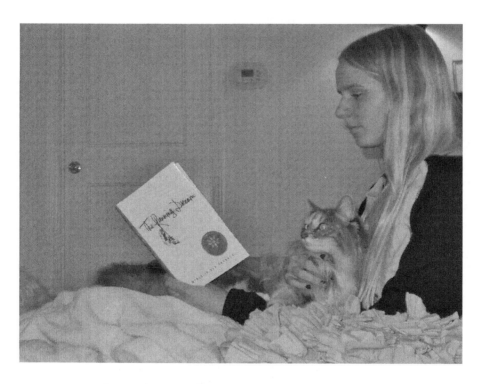

*Jacqueline reading on the couch with our cat.*

Sure, I've heard about it, learned in biology class how the cells develop, and have known some people who've been diagnosed with the disease, but I never thought it would affect us. Not our family. Not my perfect little world.

June 13, 2013. A day I don't think our mom, sister and I will ever be able to forget. Jacqueline and I came home from school - happy the day was over and we could rest a little before starting our homework — but something was up.

Our mom called us into the back living room, and asked us both to sit on the bright red couch.

She looked pained, worried, but strong. And then it came. Like a ton of bricks. That evil word. *Cancer.*

The first thing that came to my mind was *no, no this is not happening. No.* No one said anything. My lips were unable to form words. We just hugged and hugged for a while.

Then our mom, in her strongest voice asked, "Do you have any questions?" She told us about how they found a tumor in her esophagus and how she had a rare form of cancer that has a poor prognosis. Chemotherapy and radiation would start soon.

It didn't seem real. *Chemotherapy and radiation and cancer — those are things that other people go through, not us,* I thought.

I finally mustered up the strength to say, "What do we do now?" I couldn't think of what would come next. This was supposed to be our summer to relax. The one where we stayed at home, helped my grandma and rewarded ourselves for getting through the struggle that is high school.

I would be going off to college in a few months — not terribly far away but still far enough and I didn't want to leave our mom. Not now — actually not ever, but especially not now.

My mom, sister and I were a team. Everything we do, we do together. We support each other.

When it came time for college applications, my mom and sister lovingly read over my essays and made suggestions — devoting our winter break to trying to get me into college.

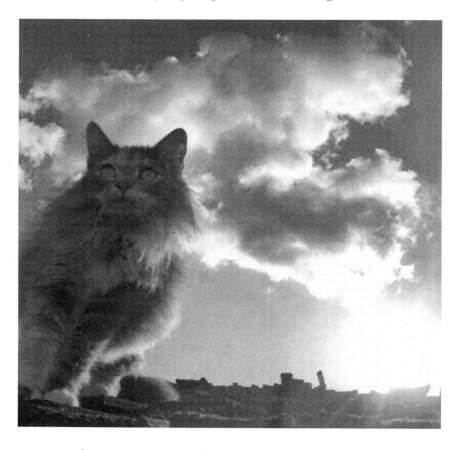

*Our cat was a comfort and a nice distraction for us during the cancer news and treatments.*

And it was successful. I got into the college of my choice. But how could I go now? I didn't want to go. Didn't want to leave. The moment she told me the diagnosis I was dead set on never leaving her side ever.

I've always thought of our mom as strong. Stronger than anyone I know. She successfully raised two teenage daughters all by herself, and made us feel like we weren't missing out on anything.

She couldn't leave us and we wouldn't let her. It was then that we all agreed — we would kick this cancer and make it through.

People survive all the time and this time our mom would be one of them. I was determined.

# WHIRLWIND OF CANCER

Cancer treatment can be fast-paced.

In our mom's case, her diagnosis was June 13, 2013; chemotherapy and radiation were the summer of 2013 (July, August), and surgery was September 30, 2013.

She had two rounds of chemotherapy with two types of chemo drugs, five weekly radiation treatments for five weeks, followed by about six weeks of recovery and then an eight-hour surgery to remove her esophagus.

While the recovery from surgery was slow, in the beginning everything occurred at lightning speed and we had to bring our A game to make it through.

From the time the word cancer comes off the doctor's lips, you and your parent will be transported by a whirlwind of doctor's appointments. Once our mom was diagnosed, she was assigned a case manager who served as a kind of middle-person between our mom and the doctors.

The case manager set up the chemotherapy, radiation and the rest of the treatment plan for our mom's case. Since the treatment plan would also include surgery, our family spent a lot of time researching the best surgeon and facility for this to take place.

All of this was occurring right after high school. With barely a high school diploma in hand, I became our mother's right-hand person. I went to almost every doctor appointment, consultation, and CT and PET scan that summer. I found notebooks to be my best friend.

Jacqueline was on a swim team that had practices sometimes twice a day and swim meets most Saturdays. I had a driver's license and she was only 14, so I drove our mom to most of the chemo and radiation appointments and Jacqueline got everything squared away at home for our mom's care.

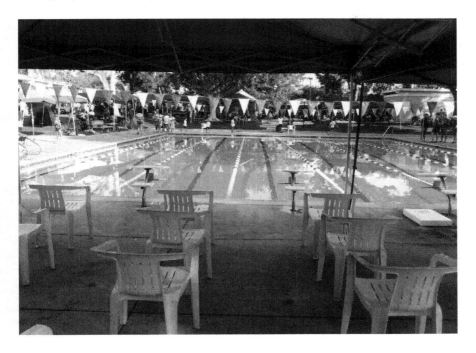

*Jacqueline could walk to the daily swim team practices while Katherine drove her mom to chemo and radiation.*

There were so many things going on at once regarding our mom's cancer care and we didn't want to mess anything up. So we wrote everything down. During doctor's visits and consultation, I took copious notes on everything that was said. It proved invaluable when we later wanted to recall what was said and didn't want to rely on memory alone.

I also love to organize. I made binders filled with all the research my family did about esophageal cancer. From WebMD and the Wikipedia page to scientific articles on PubMed to our mom's visit summaries from the doctors, the binders had everything carefully labeled.

This helped our mom when she wanted to find a specific result from a doctor's appointment or statistic from a study. We also annotated everything we put in the binder, so when we looked back we could remember what our initial thoughts were.

# TYPE OF CANCER – ESOPHAGEAL

Our mom's diagnosis was cancer of the esophagus. I had learned in school what the esophagus was—a hollow tube, about nine inches long, that connects the throat to the stomach, but I had never heard that someone could have cancer of the esophagus.

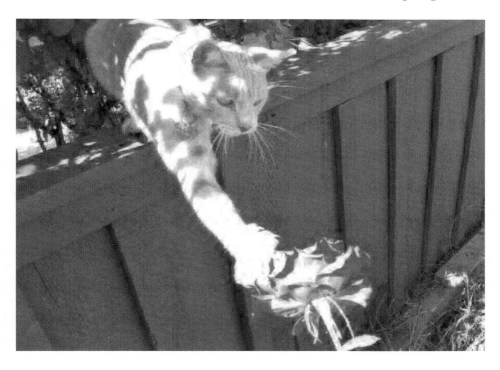

*Our cat likes roses. We were home a lot dealing with cancer, but we still enjoyed spending time with our pets.*

It's a rare cancer. Nationwide, only about 3,000 women and 16,000 men a year get it. The disease is more common in older men who smoke or drink a lot of alcohol. Our mother did not fit any of those descriptions.

The usual symptoms are heartburn and trouble swallowing food. While no cancer is good to get, esophageal cancer is one of the worst. It often has a poor prognosis. Only 15 percent of patients diagnosed with the disease will live five years.

Our mom was having some problems swallowing so she went to the doctor to have her throat checked out. Her primary physician referred her to a specialist to have a physical exam of her throat, followed by a barium swallow, which tested how she swallowed.

When the barium swallow indicated she might have a tumor, she had an endoscopy in which the physician looked down her throat and took pictures of her esophagus from the inside. He also did a biopsy, which showed the tumor was cancerous. Later she had an ultrasound, PET scan and CT scan to see how far the tumor had spread.

She had stage 3 cancer. The tumor had grown into the wall of her esophagus and into a lymph node. Fortunately, it had not spread to other parts of her body.

# RADIATION TREATMENTS

When it came time for radiation, I was in the driver's seat, literally. Since I had recently gotten my driver's license, I could drive our mom to and from her radiation appointments — a 50-minute drive by freeway. Since it was a long drive and our mom was exhausted from all the treatment and doctor's appointments, it helped a lot that I could drive her.

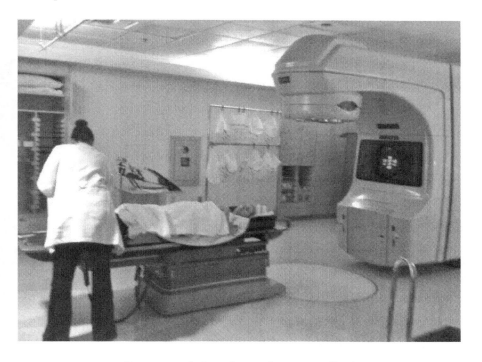

*Our mom lying flat to have a radiation treatment in the machine on the right.*

While there were shuttles that transported patients, our mom and I appreciated the time we got to spend together during that 50-minute drive on the open road. And on those rare days when our mom was too tired to stay awake for the drive, I was happy to drive with a sleeping mom beside me.

Once we arrived, I sat in the waiting room, with all the other friends and family, for about 15 minutes, while our mom received her radiation treatment. We went to radiation about five times a week for five weeks. Radiation sessions were more frequent than chemotherapy, but each session was much shorter in duration.

# CHEMOTHERAPY TREATMENTS

I also accompanied our mom to her chemo appointments. Before the initial session of sitting in the chair with the chemo drugs injected in the veins, we had to watch a 30-minute video about what chemo is, how it affects the body, and what to do if something goes wrong. We weren't warned about the PICC line, but I'll go into more detail about that later.

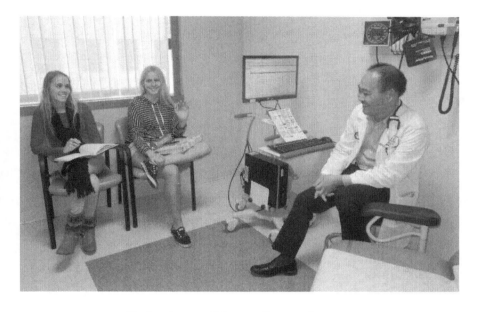

*Katherine and Jacqueline took notes at*
*their mother's oncology appointment.*

Chemotherapy is weird. And it's long. Your parent will sit in this big recliner—which is similar to a La-Z-Boy chair but with plastic sterile material. A nurse will come in with a big sterile gown and gloves and insert the needle connected to the chemotherapy into your parent's arm. And that's all they do. Then you wait. And wait. It's best to bring something to do.

Our mom and I would pack books to read, snacks and her laptop to pass the time. We also naturally can just talk to each other for a long time—like we do on long car rides— so just chatting as the medicine dripped away was also a nice way to pass the time.

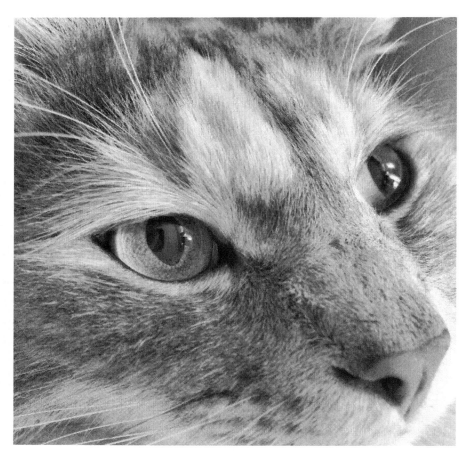

*When our mom was on chemo her doctor told her to stay away from our pets when she was more susceptible to infection.*

After the PICC line removal, our mom's arm turned bright red, swelled up and she started having trouble breathing. The chemo head nurse told us to go to the emergency room. After an ultrasound and a few other tests, the doctors found out she had a deep vein thrombosis (DVT) and substantial blood clots in the lung, or a pulmonary embolism (PE).

This can be deadly, which I didn't know about until after we were in the clear so I didn't worry too much initially. It just goes to show that sometimes the treatment can be a real danger, and you have to prepare for whatever cancer, and treatments throw at you.

Recovering from a pulmonary embolism is a slow process. Our mom had to regain her lung function and take baby steps every day to build up her ability to walk or stand. It took a while, (and even now her lungs don't work at 100 percent capacity) but her lungs held up for the surgery, which is what really mattered.

# CONSULTATIONS WITH FOUR SURGEONS

Since our mom had such a rare cancer, not a lot of doctors were familiar with this form of cancer. The local surgeons under our mom's insurance plan who had performed esophagectomies did not do them very frequently.

So we set off on a mission to find the best surgeon for our mom. The surgery is very risky and invasive — in our mom's case involving three incisions, from six to eight inches in length, on the neck, belly and back to remove the esophagus and half of the stomach. (Although minimally invasive surgery, in which the incisions are smaller, is available, our mother was not a candidate for this surgery because of the risks associated with her pulmonary embolism.)

After the esophagus and half the stomach are removed, the remaining half of the stomach is turned into a new esophagus and is connected to her throat near her neck. Her food then goes directly to her small intestine. Since her stomach (now her esophagus) is larger than her old esophagus, it pushes against her lungs a little and gives a different sensation. But it works.

The mortality rate from the surgery is about five percent and we wanted to do everything we could to have our mom be in the winning percentage. We had consultations with four thoracic surgeons who performed esophagectomies and discussed each of their plans for the surgery. They all had different opinions and approaches.

Here the binders and notebooks came in handy, as we could look back at all four surgery plans to determine the best option.

In the end, we went with the surgeon who had performed the most esophagectomies and had the best survival rate, even though he was outside of our mom's original insurance plan.

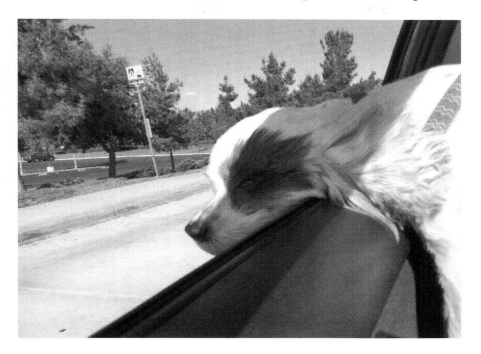

*Our dog loves car rides, but didn't get
to go on the rides to the hospital.*

.

If your current insurance plan does not have physicians who provide the services you require, you can request a referral to a different doctor. If your insurance company denies the referral, you can file a grievance and then later an appeal with the insurance plan and an appeal with your state. This was an added challenge for us and we helped our mom with all the paperwork. We felt the very best medical care was required based on the life-threatening aspects of this surgery.

We were lucky that our mom had a friend who was a gastroenterologist who referred her to an outstanding thoracic surgeon, as our mom did a lot of research online and it was still difficult to find the most qualified surgeon online. She looked at the *U.S. News & World Report* Top Hospital Rankings and The LeapFrog Hospital Group as a good starting point, but it was hard to find the exact details she wanted. She was looking for a surgeon who had performed this particular surgery a large number of times, with low mortality rates.

For this type of surgery, there is a published report indicating that in some hospitals 25 percent of patients die within 30 days of the surgery. The surgeon our mom went to had not had a patient die within 30 days of the surgery for three years prior to when he operated on her. She felt confident with him doing the surgery to remove her esophagus, half her stomach and 77 lymph nodes

It is always good to get second, third or even fourth opinions if you're not totally confident with your surgeon. We felt our mom was in the best hands she could be in and now, over two years after the surgery, she is doing well — although she still has some challenges — but most importantly, she is still alive.

# COMPLEMENTARY TREATMENTS

Along with the medical treatment that the doctor ordered, our mom looked into complementary treatments. Complementary treatments mean treatments in *addition* to conventional medical treatment. This is not to be confused with alternative treatment, which is a treatment used *instead* of traditional treatment.

Our family was determined to do everything we could to defeat the cancer. We researched many complementary treatments and our mom tried everything that didn't seem dangerous. From our research, we found physical, mental, spiritual and emotional treatments.

## PHYSICAL COMPLEMENTARY TREATMENTS

Our mom started by changing her diet. Websites and books suggest different types of diets to fight off cancer, but the one we found recommended most often, with the best chance of survival, was a vegan diet.

Vegan is similar to a vegetarian diet, in that you don't eat meat, but you also don't eat any animal products. Animal products include meat, but also milk or eggs — anything from an animal. Most of the time our mom is a vegan.

During the radiation treatment, we had to puree most of her food because her throat really hurt and she could barely swallow water.

She also has cut back on sugar and sweets because research we found said that sugar feeds the cancer. In fact, how a PET scan works is that the patient drinks a glucose, or sugar drink, with a radioactive marker. The glucose will collect in regions of the body where cancer is present because cancer tumors have a high rate of glucose metabolism and therefore these regions appear as hot spots on the PET scan.

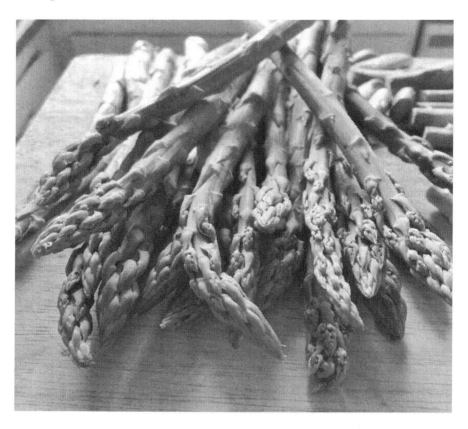

*We started eating more vegetables, which most of the books we read indicated were helpful to patients who were recovering from cancer.*

Organic food was also highly recommended from our research. While it is more expensive than regular food, organic food is said to be better because it theoretically doesn't have chemicals from pesticides that can cause cancer. Our mom also tried juicing, eating lots of vegetables, and making plant protein powder shakes.

She started every morning with organic oatmeal to which she added hemp, chia seeds, flax seeds, raisins and ginger water — all organic when possible. She would add some fresh fruit too, sometimes.

She is more of a grazer than a cook, so during the day she ate natural unprocessed foods most of the time, such as raw unsalted nuts, avocados, quinoa and beans. She ate a banana every day (because they were soft) and ate lots of fruits and vegetables. Sometimes if we were going out for dinner, she would eat fish or shrimp.

Aside from food, our mom tried to keep her body active and stress-free. We went on walks around our neighborhood and watched yoga. Our mom didn't always have the energy or inclination to do much of the actual yoga but she found just watching the DVDs to be relaxing — so that was better than nothing.

Our mom also had massages, which were recommended to her by an esophageal cancer survivor. She had Googled "who lived the longest with esophageal cancer" and found a man named Ed Mitchell who had survived 18 years after esophageal cancer and offered to help anyone with the disease. He shared his story, and told people what worked for him and how he survived. She followed pretty much everything he recommended.

In addition to tips on eating, exercise, getting the best physicians and laughter, he recommended daily self-massage and weekly massages from a massage therapist, based on the Ayurveda treatment. While we couldn't find a local Ayurveda center that was available, we researched the approach and our mom had massages whenever possible.

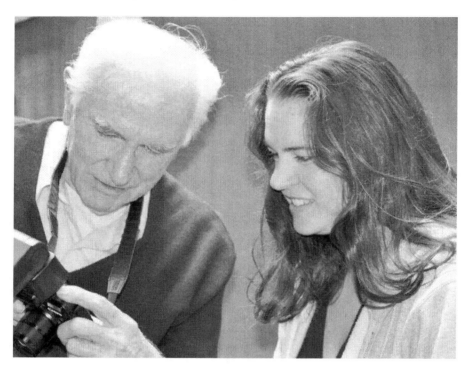

*Ed Mitchell was a long-time esophageal cancer survivor who encouraged cancer patients and inspired our mom to believe that she could survive. He is seen here with his daughter Katherine.*

## MENTAL, SPIRITUAL & EMOTIONAL COMPLEMENTARY TREATMENTS

Besides physical strength, a lot of mental and emotional stamina is needed to fight cancer. Our family would pray together before her exams and surgery. We prayed that there wouldn't be any problems and for a cancer free result.

Our mom also looked into hypnotherapy, healing, and meditation DVDs. She had a personalized hypnotherapy audio tape that she listened to before her surgery to ease her mind and make her feel confident in what was to come.

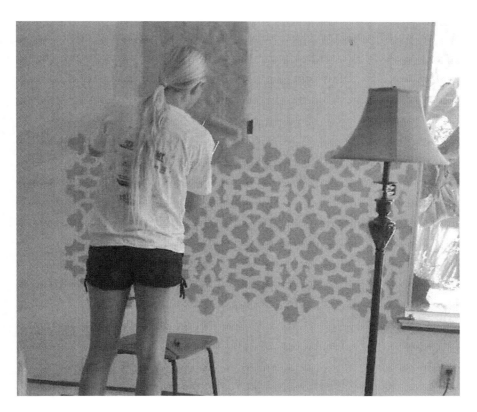

*Jacqueline painted the living room wall*
*to make our house more cheerful.*

Many cancer patients also try a therapist or psychiatric consultation. While our family didn't do this much, as we were more focused on getting rid of the cancer than talking about our feelings toward the cancer, it can be a good option to look into if you and your parent want to open up to someone about the challenges your parent is facing with cancer.

You can also confide in family, friends, and Internet cancer support groups. Many hospitals have support groups where your parent can go to talk to other patients with the same cancer. Because our mom's cancer was so rare, we couldn't find any local groups.

Our mom had a couple of very good friends she talked to regularly about her treatments, and they both came down to help us during the surgery. Our next-door neighbor was a huge help in getting us food and in driving us to the airport and to doctor's appointments when I wasn't available.

Our mom found out about a website called CancerCompass after she had gone through the hardest parts of her cancer battle, but now goes on the website to provide advice and support to those with esophageal cancer who are still at earlier stages of their cancer treatment.

We also wanted to make our house more cheerful, so Jacqueline picked out a stencil and some bright yellow paint and in one day painted an entire wall in our living room in a fun pattern. We also got four bright yellow cushions to match. This really brightened our mom's spirits and made us all happier!

# RESULTS OF CHEMOTHERAPY, RADIATION & COMPLEMENTARY TREATMENTS

Before your parent starts chemotherapy and radiation, the doctor might tell you and your parent how likely it is that the cancer tumor will respond to treatment. Our mom's oncologist told her that 20 percent of patients with esophageal cancer had a full response to the radiation and chemotherapy treatment, meaning there was no sign of cancer afterward.

Another 20 percent had no response; the tumor had not shrunk from the treatment. The remaining 60 percent had some response, so the tumor size was reduced but some cancer remained.

CT scans and PET scans are used to visualize the cancer.

After our mom's treatment, the scans showed a complete response, or no sign of cancer. Even though this was great news and we felt like we could breathe a sigh of relief, the cancer could still be there.

Our mom's doctors explained and very strongly stressed that there could still be cancer cells in the body because cancer would have to be about the size of a marble to show up on the scans. Anything smaller would not be picked up by the scans.

Therefore, after much internal struggle on our mom's part, as she really didn't want to have the surgery, we decided to go ahead with surgery to remove the esophagus just in case there was some small remnants of cancer in her esophagus.

If we were not as aggressive with this treatment, and there was some cancer left, it could spread and metastasize and we would be in a much worse situation.

# LEAVING FOR COLLEGE
# TWO WEEKS BEFORE SURGERY

With helping our mom with radiation and chemotherapy and their aftereffects, as well as helping her prepare for surgery, it's safe to say that the last thing on my mind was starting college. I would be far away, about 400 miles, in a city I wasn't familiar with.

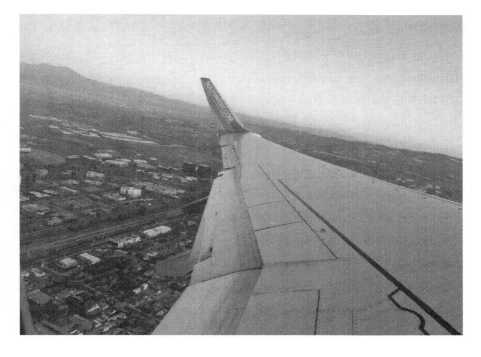

*Katherine spent all summer helping her mom through chemo, radiation and a pulmonary embolism, then left to start college two weeks before the surgery.*

On top of that, I had never really been away from home, other than an overnight sleepover, so this was uncharted territory for me. But most important is I would be studying in a dorm room rather than helping my cancer-stricken mom at home.

Our mom always thinks of everyone else, though. She was determined not to have the cancer affect my ability to go to college. So I went. She couldn't go with me to get me settled into college because she was still weak from the pulmonary embolism and it wasn't a good idea for her to travel.

I took a flight up north. A family friend met me at the airport when I arrived and helped me buy a bike and some other college supplies. Our mom had already bought a small microwave, small refrigerator and printer for my room that she shipped to our friend's house, so we were as organized as we could be. We loaded up her truck and off I went to college!

Our friend helped me unpack, met my roommate, and attended the convocation or opening college events for families — some people thought she was my mom and she certainly stepped up, filled in and made my first days at college the best they could be.

I did my best to put on a happy face with the rest of the excited college freshmen. But I missed my mom.

The good news was that I would see her soon. Less than two weeks after starting college, I flew home to be with her the day before her surgery.

I missed a few days of college, which wasn't ideal considering I was just starting the school year and just starting college, but it was all worth it to be with our mom for such an important procedure - it could save her life.

After the surgery, I came home almost every weekend of my first quarter to help take care of our mom as she was recovering, and to give Jacqueline a break as she was our mom's full-time caregiver and she had just turned 15.

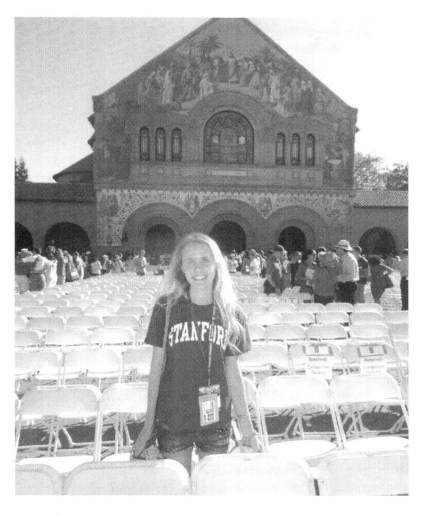

*Katherine at her first day of college of her freshman year.*
*Two weeks after her classes started, she went home to help her*
*mom through surgery and missed a few days of classes.*

The lighter college load made this a lot easier and while it was still hard juggling everything even with fewer classes, it would have been next to impossible with a heavier course load.

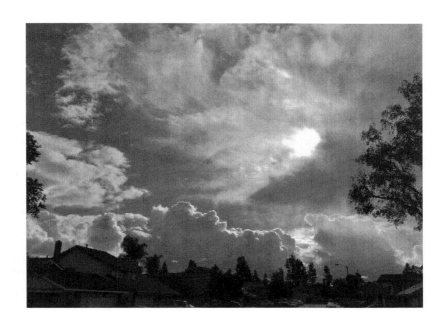

# OUR ROAD MAP –
# SURGERY TO RECOVERY

By
JACQUELINE CARR
*Age 14-15 at time of mother's cancer*

## PREPARING FOR SURGERY

September 29th. My 15th birthday, aka the night before our mom's surgery. We celebrated with a dinner and birthday cake at our next-door neighbors' house.

It was bittersweet celebrating and having fun knowing that in less than 24 hours would be the day that we had been preparing for all along—surgery day.

My birthday party celebration was a good distraction from thinking about the surgery and eased the tension that we all felt.

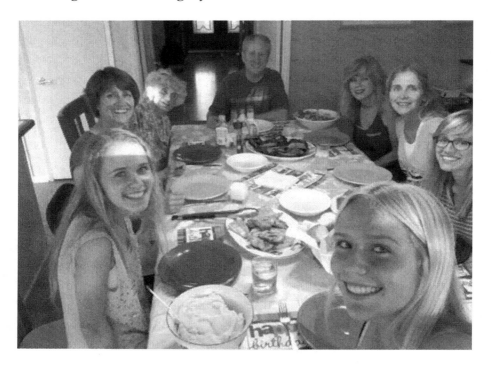

*Dinner with friends and family the night before surgery helped us get our mind off what was to come.*

The next morning we got up very early and left at about 2:30 in the morning to drive an hour to Los Angeles for a 4:00 a.m. check in. Our mom's good friend flew into town the night before to go with us to the hospital.

There was no traffic at that time in the morning — rare for a drive to Los Angeles — and it was quiet and we were all a little groggy still.

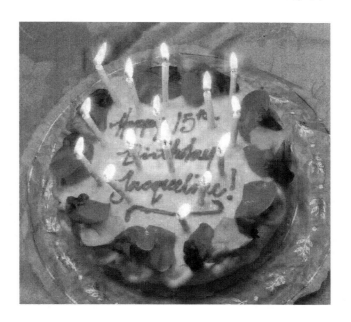

*Blowing out candles the night before surgery.*

# SURGERY

When we checked in at the hospital for our mom's surgery, the nurse told our mom that only one person could go into the pre-op room with her. So Katherine and our mom were rushed away to pre-op and said goodbye before I was really ready.

But they sent video messages from the pre-op room so we could still be in touch. Our mom was very calm and cheerful. She had prepared emotionally for the surgery through a hypno-therapist who had created a CD just for the surgery day.

I found out later that when she was on the gurney in pre-op, she was happy that a heater went inside her paper gown to keep her warm and toasty. After chemo and with her weight loss she always got very cold.

Katherine said they met the nurses, anesthesiologist and surgeon and everything went very smoothly.

Our mom had an IV and an epidural shot in her back and Katherine watched everything while I waited with our mom's friend.

Then they wheeled our mom off to the operating room and Katherine joined our mom's friend and me for the long wait — which the surgeon said would be at least eight hours.

Lots of waiting.

I grouped a couple of chairs together and made a fort in the middle of the hospital waiting room, knowing that I would probably stay longer than anyone else would. I had packed clothes and homework for a weeklong stay and Katherine was just going to be there for a few days.

I had arranged with my teachers and the administration at my high school to take a week off from school and was going to basically live in the Intensive Care Unit (ICU) with our mom while my sister went back to college.

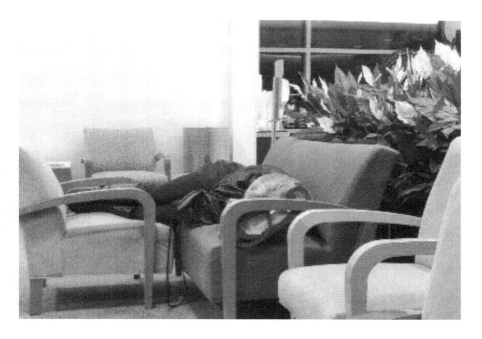

*Sleeping in the hospital waiting room.*

Our mom had two good friends who would also keep an eye on things at the hospital — just in case something took a turn for the worse. One friend stayed at a nearby hotel the first week and then our mom's other good friend — her cousin — came down for the second week and then to drive our mom home. (I was 15 and didn't have a license yet.)

The day of her surgery, I saw the sunrise while waiting in the hospital lobby. I would be inside that hospital all day, even as the sun was setting.

Time just seemed to be a blur, blended together yet so distinct and stagnant.

I would occasionally ask the front desk people how much longer it would be. We tried to be as calm as possible. The other doctors would often come out and talk to other families about how the surgeries for their loved ones went.

We were excited to finally hear the news that our mom was out of the operating room, as the surgery took a little longer than the eight hours that was expected.

I quickly packed up my belongings and headed to a private room to talk with the surgeon.

We were concerned about whether our mom's lung with the pulmonary embolism could withstand the surgery, as her good lung was deflated during the surgery so the esophagus could be removed. The bad lung had to function on its own for eight hours.

After the surgery, we met with the surgeon who was very reassuring. He said something along the lines of, "We took out the esophagus. She's in the recovery room. You can go up there shortly."

We were overjoyed.

Katherine asked, "How did the lung do?"

He said, "It held up." We thanked him profusely and then he left.

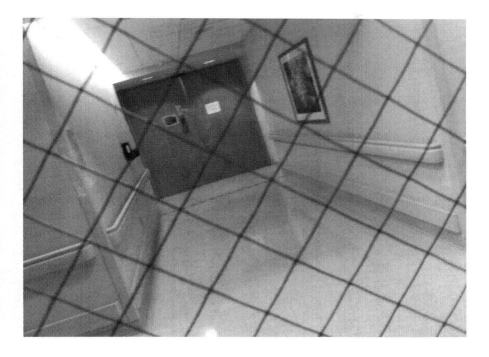

*The view from the waiting room to the ICU –*
*Jacqueline and Katherine waited for eight hours*
*to see their mother after surgery.*

Then we went upstairs to yet again another waiting room on the level of the ICU.

While people were bent over sleeping on upright chairs and others were crying while a soccer game hummed in the background on a TV, I stood there, anxiously peering through the glass whenever I heard a hospital bed being wheeled down the hallway and into the corridors of the ICU section.

One after another, I waited like a dog looking for his master in a crowded dog park. I waited for our mother.

When her hospital bed finally turned the corner, I was happy that she was alive, but I was surprised at the amount of people hovering around her and the complicated hospital equipment strewn around her.

When I finally saw our mom up close, she was big and puffy. She could barely open her eyes. There were tubes sticking out everywhere and beeping machines. There were tubes in her nose and her neck. She could barely talk.

The TV was blaring and all I could think about was our mom.

Our mom smiled and said, "Yeah, we did it." That was the first thing she said to us.

We saw our mom for about five minutes and then we had to leave because it was emotionally too intense to handle.

Katherine wanted to leave because she said she wanted to throw up. I started to cry.

Katherine said she had a physical response and that her body wanted to throw up because it's our mom who we have known our whole entire life, and who has pretty much always looked the same.

And now her cheeks were three times their size, her eyes were like little small buttons pushed in her face and she didn't seem like the person we'd left eight hours before.

So we left after a few minutes to try to compose ourselves and the nurse found us and said that our mom wanted to see us.

So we came back to the room with our mom.

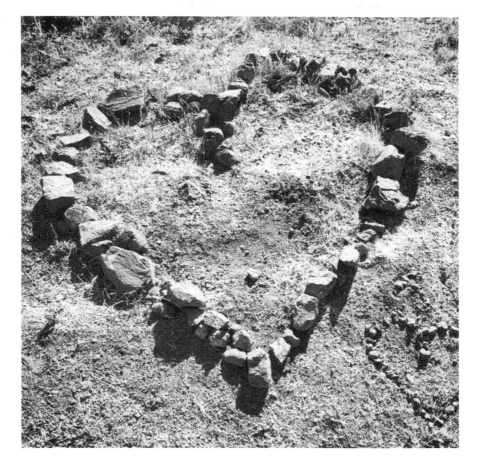

*Although times might be rough, you have to be there*
*for your parent because your parent needs you.*

Our mom did not know there were tubes in her nose and she put her hand up to her face and tried to swat them off.

Our mom tried to hold our hands and be really nice to us.

She was like sadly sweet. She said, "How are you girls? Did you get something to eat?" and then she'd fall asleep because she was heavily medicated.

She was on so many drugs she wasn't like herself.

She had a high squeaky voice and couldn't say much.

I didn't think she would want to see what she looked like, so when she asked for a mirror after a couple of days I said I couldn't find one. The nurse said she was pumped with saline and that's why she was so puffy.

After a few days, her face wasn't as puffy and we took the only picture we have of just her with all the machines around her in the hospital during her stay.

During the surgery, the surgeon made three big incisions. Our mom had two drainage tubes in her belly, tubes in her nose, chest, and back and an IV in her arm. She also had a feeding tube coming out of her small intestine. She was connected to a lot of machines.

# HELPING IN THE ICU

Katherine flew down from college for the surgery and took a few days off from the start of her college. We both slept in our mom's room in the ICU.

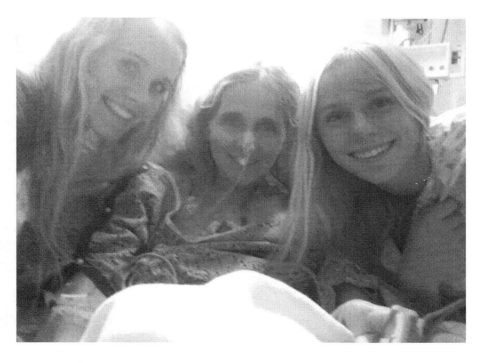

*After a few days in the ICU our mom was feeling a little better and smiled with us for a picture — although she still had the annoying tube in her nose.*

Our mom was in the hospital for ten days — seven of those were in the ICU. About half of the people who have her type of surgery have some sort of complication — some are serious and some are minor. The average hospital stay is 10 days, but those people who have complications can stay 40 days or more.

Because the surgery was risky, it would be hard on our mom. As a family, we decided that I would stay with our mom for seven days, and Katherine would stay when she could.

Although we were both very busy with school and Katherine was just starting college, we felt our mom really needed us and that it would help her recovery if we were there to help her.

At one point our mom said she could handle it by herself and she didn't need us to be there, but looking back on it I know it would have been much harder for her, and she really appreciated our help.

Each day when she was in the hospital, she had different challenges and milestones that she had to reach.

At first, it was excruciatingly painful for her to even get out of bed and sit in the chair. She was on very strong pain medication and could not move very much.

Every day she had x-rays of her lungs to make sure she wasn't getting pneumonia, and a technician came twice a day for her to do breathing exercises.

Our mom had an eight-inch cut on her back. The surgeon deflated her right lung and cut her ribs during the operation so the he could remove her esophagus through her back. He also removed half her stomach and 77 lymph nodes. He made a six-inch incision on her neck, so he could attach what was left of her esophagus to the other half of her stomach.

The surgeon converted her stomach into a tube that worked like an esophagus so our mom could still eat. The food went to

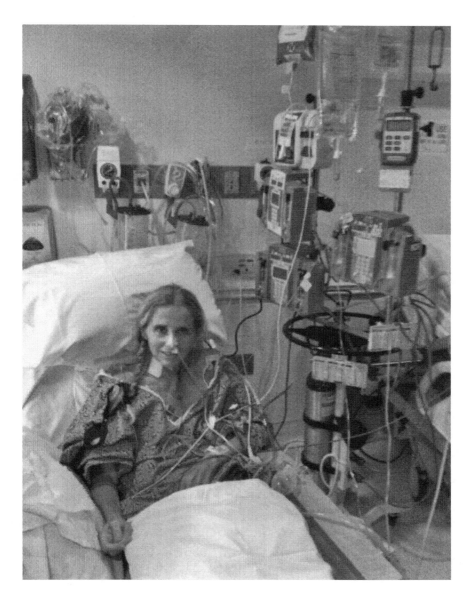

*Our mom had nine tubes coming out of her after the eight-hour surgery to remove her esophagus.*

her small intestine straight through the new tube. She wouldn't have a functioning stomach after the surgery and would have life-long adjustments in her eating. But it was worth it to her because she had such a deadly cancer and this was the best chance for survival.

She also had a seven-inch cut on her belly, which allowed the surgeons access to accomplish this high risk, complicated but lifesaving surgery.

After the surgery, she had to practice breathing with an incentive spirometer — which was a small plastic device with a little ball in it that she had to raise by inhaling into the device. Her doctor wanted her to get up to 1500 ml in the incentive spirometer, and we encouraged her to practice regularly and kept charts on this so she wouldn't forget.

She had various daily tests to see how she was progressing.

Each day we would meet with the surgeon who had interns and nurses with him, and they would review her progress. We kept our mom on track and encouraged her to do all the things the doctor requested, even though she didn't feel like it because she was in so much pain and her brain wasn't working very well because of all the pain medicine.

The doctor rounds were always something that my sister and I anticipated daily. The rounds mean that the surgeon, interns and nurses would all walk into our mom's small ICU room with their wheeling computers and handheld note pads and they would fill the doctor in on our mom's condition and her numbers.

The surgeon would then quickly state what he thought should be improving and what he thought was working well. Because the doctor rounds were typically very quick and there wasn't much time to ponder questions, our mom would have us write down any concerns or questions on her white board so when he came in we would have all our questions ready.

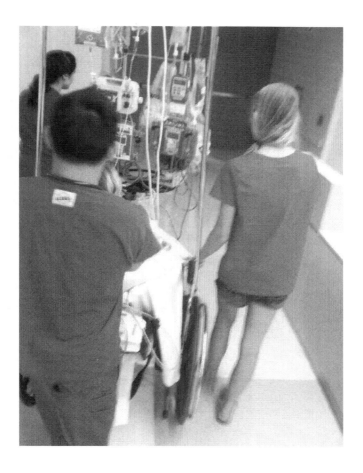

*Katherine, right, walking down the hall with our mom in the wheelchair, with all equipment for a test.*

We appreciated the surgeon, the nurses, and the staff and tried to show it. We brought a box of See's candy and it was put next to the nurses' station. In a few minutes, it was all gone and we realized we should have bought two boxes!

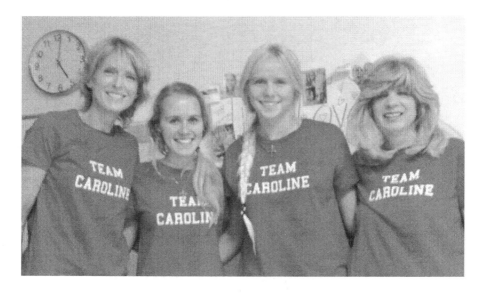

*Our mom's cousin, left, and her*
*friend, right joined us in the ICU.*

Our mom's cousin had designed and ordered about 20 shirts that were bright blue and said "TEAM CAROLINE." She had them delivered and we all wore them — even our mom's surgeon wore one as well as some of the interns and nurses.

It made us feel that we were all on the same team trying to help our mom and it reminded me of when I was on soccer, swim and baseketball teams, and when I rowed for a year. When I was on teams, we all had a lot of team spirit and were very competitive.

At the hospital, we all wanted our mom to recover from the surgery without complications and to go home as soon as she could, and we were her biggest cheerleaders.

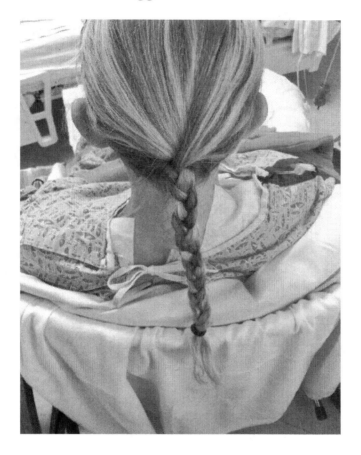

*Jacqueline braided our mom's hair*
*when she was in the hospital.*

We made a sign that said, "We Love You Mommy" and "You Are So Strong" and hung it on the wall with pictures of our family and pets. It cheered our mom in the hospital.
ack up.

Just like our mom cheered me on for all the years she went to my games and swim meets, I was cheering her on and encouraging her to inhale through the breathing machine, take a bite of food, move into the chair or try to walk. I brushed and braided her hair just like she brushed and braided my hair when I was a little girl.

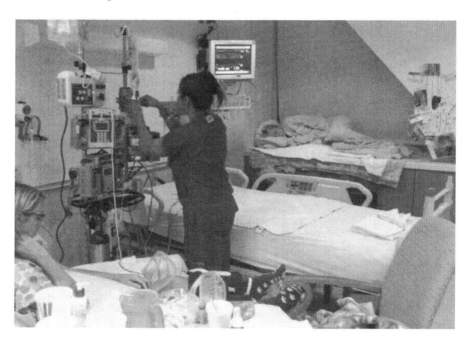

*Jacqueline is seen sleeping on the windowsill ledge, far right, of her mother's ICU room.*

Katherine slept on a reclining chair and I slept on a windowsill ledge. Not ideal, but we wanted to be with her and didn't want to go to the hotel with our mom's friend.

I acted as our mom's room nurse, adjusting her pillows, brushing her hair and keeping track of the numbers on a big monitor right above my windowsill bed. If something unusual happened that looked like it needed the nurse's attention, I would alert the nurse.

There was one set of nurses during the day and another set at night. Each time they would change shifts they wrote their names on the white board in our mom's room.

It was hard to transition between one nurse and the other because I would get comfortable with one nurse and before I knew it, I would be hearing one nurse filling in another before their shift ended.

# HOMEWORK IN THE ICU

In order to take a week off from school I was on an independent contract. I gathered my homework from my teachers and filled the requirements needed to miss a week of school.

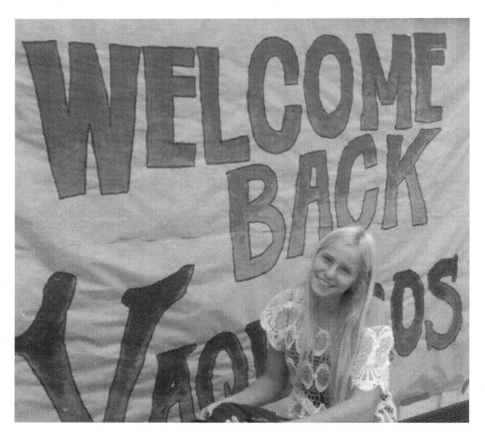

*Jacqueline's first day of 10th grade. She later packed up her school books and moved into the ICU for a week.*

I set up a little bed of pillows and hospital blankets on a small hard-surfaced windowsill — my workplace.

I did my homework, typed emails, talked on the phone and occasionally ate in a two- by four-foot section of a room perched above the ground. Our mom often didn't want to smell the food I had so I often ate outside in the waiting room.

It was hard to juggle my schoolwork with caring for our mom, since I would always think that our mom was teetering on a life and death situation while my schoolwork would always be there.

It was hard to concentrate on learning flash cards of Spanish words while also watching over our mom and monitoring all the beeping and blinking monitor lights.

It was hard to come to terms with my sister leaving to go back to college because I knew that once we got home I would be our mom's primary caregiver — although she was trying to line up professional caregivers and our mom's cousin stayed with us for the first week.

# CAREGIVING AT HOME

Our mom's cousin drove her back from the hospital and helped around the house a lot while we transitioned to our new life. She helped our mom fill her prescriptions and bought groceries. She was a very positive, bouncy person and she did everything enthusiastically. She also bought devices to help our mom, such as a chair seat for the shower and other equipment that we hadn't anticipated she would need.

When our mom came home from the hospital, she had two drainage tubes in her belly that collected the excess fluid. They were about the size of small grenades and we had to empty them a few times a day and measure how much fluid was in them. She also had a feeding tube coming out of her belly and we had to connect it to the feeding tube machine every night.

I think we were a little apprehensive when our mom got home from the hospital because we were used to getting all the help from the nurses and we were concerned that we wouldn't know what to do if something went wrong.

Our mom's insurance covered some home health care so nurses were sent to our house for a quick check up every day or so in the beginning. They checked her bandages on her incisions and her vital signs.

But there was a lot more to be done than a quick check.

Because our mom was physically so weak and could barely get out of bed, I was in charge of mixing her pain medicine, preparing the feeding tube machine and emptying the drains that protruded from her abdomen.

I moved my bed into the living room so that I could be right next to our mom's room in case something was to happen.

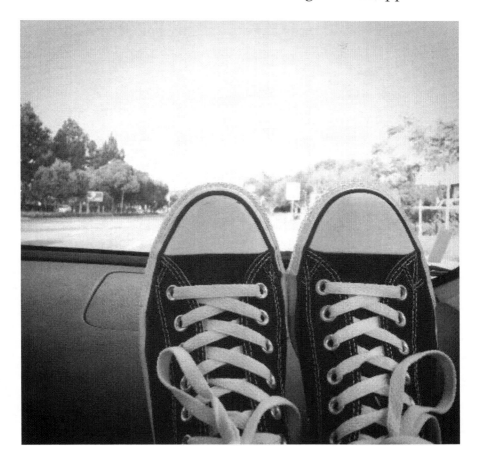

*Being your parent's primary caregiver won't leave you with many free moments so put your feet up when you can.*

I also had to sleep very lightly as if she was a newborn baby.

Ideally, it is good to line up some extra helpers ahead of time. We signed up with one agency that could send people to help by the hour, and we tried to find a live-in helper.

These attempts didn't prove successful and our efforts to get extra helpers was more work than it was worth. I am an overprotective and sensitive daughter; I could quickly and intuitively sense our mom's needs before she even asked for anything.

It came to the point when I was tending to our mom more during the time the agency helpers were here than when they weren't here. It also got awkward when I was busy hustling around the house and they were sitting reading a magazine on our couch as if there was nothing to do.

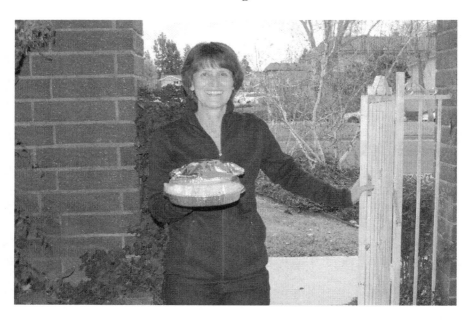

*A warm meal and a happy smile.*

I was so appreciative that our next-door neighbor brought us dinner almost every night before and after our mom's surgery.

A hot meal wrapped in tin foil can bring such happiness to a teenage girl. I would be so happy to hear the knock on the door and be greeted with a handful of food options every night!

Before our mom was sick, I cooked dinner a lot for our family, but when my days got busier, it was harder to take time out of the day to cook a meal.

Our mom was also sensitive to smells of food that she knew she couldn't eat, so it would be too tempting for me to cook a meal without giving some to our mom and then deal with the mess afterward.

When Katherine came home on the weekends it gave me about a day and a half to catch up and get ahead in my schoolwork, and take a small break from taking care of our mom.

Katherine took over the weekend shift in order to alleviate some of the pressure that had been building up during the week. It was sad having Katherine leave every Sunday night because I would miss her and I knew that I had a long week ahead full of school and taking care of our mom.

# NEW NORMAL

Our mom's recovery was slow—it was many, many months before she could function very well, and almost a year until she began to feel like herself again. At school, I kept my activities to a minimum. I had wanted to try out for the volleyball team that year but I knew I wouldn't have time. I didn't socialize as much or take on any new extracurricular activities at school.

Our mom had to adjust to a "new normal." Many of the basic tasks that we take for granted had to change—like eating, drinking and even sleeping.

During the recovery stage, our mom had a strict diet; she had to be weaned back on food after using the feeding tube for three and a half weeks. She started with soft foods that were mushy or blended, since her esophagus was taken out and the new pseudo-esophagus—made from her stomach—was a source of discomfort.

Fatigue was also a major problem. I would go to school for six hours with our mom resting on the couch, and I would come back with her being in the same position, having not moved all day.

She wasn't motivated to be active and she was always so tired and out of it. Later into her recovery, she would try and walk around our house and take small walks in the neighborhood.

Her fatigue and exhaustion went hand in hand with the invasive surgery she had undergone, along with the pulmonary embolism she had before the surgery. All of these factors limited her ability to be active and comfortable.

While today she can eat normal food—although in smaller portions with other restrictions—and walk longer distances, there is one thing that will always stay constant: her sleeping position.

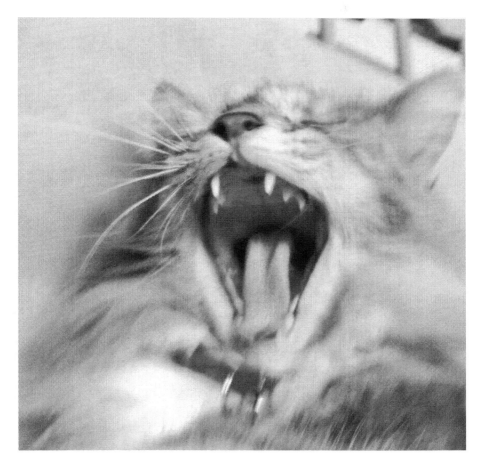

*Our mom was tired all the time and so were we.*

Our mom has to sleep at a 45-degree angle every night or else she runs the risk of having food come up or breathing it in. This is because during the operation the surgeon removed the muscle that prevents food from coming back up.

Whether it is a wedge, extra pillows or an adjustable bed, there are many methods to ensure that she is sleeping in the correct position. This sleeping position is crucial in order to avoid choking on food from her small intestine or inhaling it into her lungs. If she inhales food, she could get pneumonia or die.

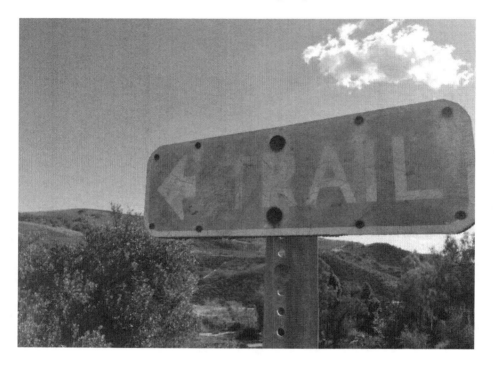

*For months after her major surgery, we just walked*
*slowly around the neighbhorhood with our mom,*
*much later, we hit the trails.*

With all of this being said, it seems like she could never have her normal life back again, and that all of these limitations would make everything a chore and hinder her — and our — happiness. We have learned to adjust and consider this lifestyle as the new normal.

Today I subconsciously know what foods don't agree with her, and also how high up she needs to sleep to avoid aspiration.

Before our mom was diagnosed with cancer, I would always wake up to the sound of brewing coffee. Now I wake up to the sound of boiling ginger water. Our mom peels and chops ginger and boils in water every morning. She drinks it throughout the day because it is high on the alkaline scale. She read in many of her cancer books that it is hard for cancer to grow in an alkaline environment.

Once our mom could start eating solids again, she tried to stay on an organic vegan diet because she read that was the best diet to avoid cancer. Although different people make different food choices, this is what she selected. She eats, fish and dairy on very rare occasions.

She has checkups, which include blood tests, a CT scan and endoscopy to look down her throat. There is a 70 percent chance of recurrence and she is very thankful to be alive. She is always happy and relieved when the scans come back but it is a little stressful for all of us while we wait for the results.

This was a very intense time for our family but it happened all within about six months. It put life into perspective for us and our schoolwork seemed insignificant compared to the life-threatening challenge our mother was facing.

Because we come from a single parent family there was no other parent who could step up and do all the things we did, so we got a real crash course in cancer care.

We looked for a book that could help us help our mom but all the books we saw were about how a parent can help a child or teen deal with the emotional aspects of a parent's cancer. Because we were very busy dealing with all the details of our mom's cancer, we didn't really have time to get depressed — although seeing her after surgery was scary.

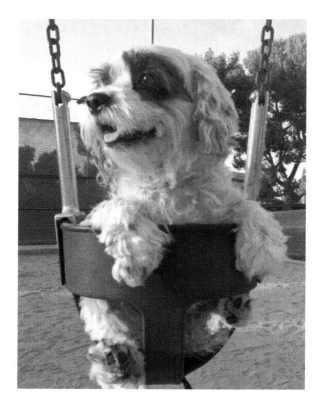

*Our dog was happy that life got more normal again and she had more walks and could play in the swing at the park again.*

Our family got very close during this ordeal and we are so thankful that she had great medical care, had the support of amazing friends, and got good results.

My birthday party celebration was a good distraction from thinking about the surgery and eased the tension that we all felt.

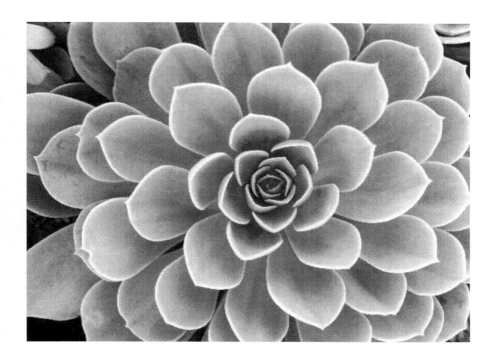

*We are now planting succulents in our garden
to help with the drought in California.*

We also kept busy doing all the things we read about in books to try to get rid of the cancer. While we don't really know if they worked or if it was the chemo, radiation and surgery — they certainly didn't hurt and it made us feel that we were taking good care of her and she was taking good care of herself.

Although we didn't focus as much on our school work, activities and social lives during the time that our mom's health was in more of a crisis mode, as her health problems settled down we got caught up on our own lives again.

It has been over two years out now since her surgery, and all tests show no sign of cancer. We need to wait five years before she can be considered cured of cancer.

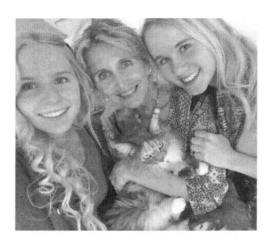

*We are happy that our mom*
*now has no signs of cancer.*

# ABCs of CANCER –
# 127 TIPS, TERMS & TIDBITS

Alarm

Alkaline

American Cancer Society

Apps

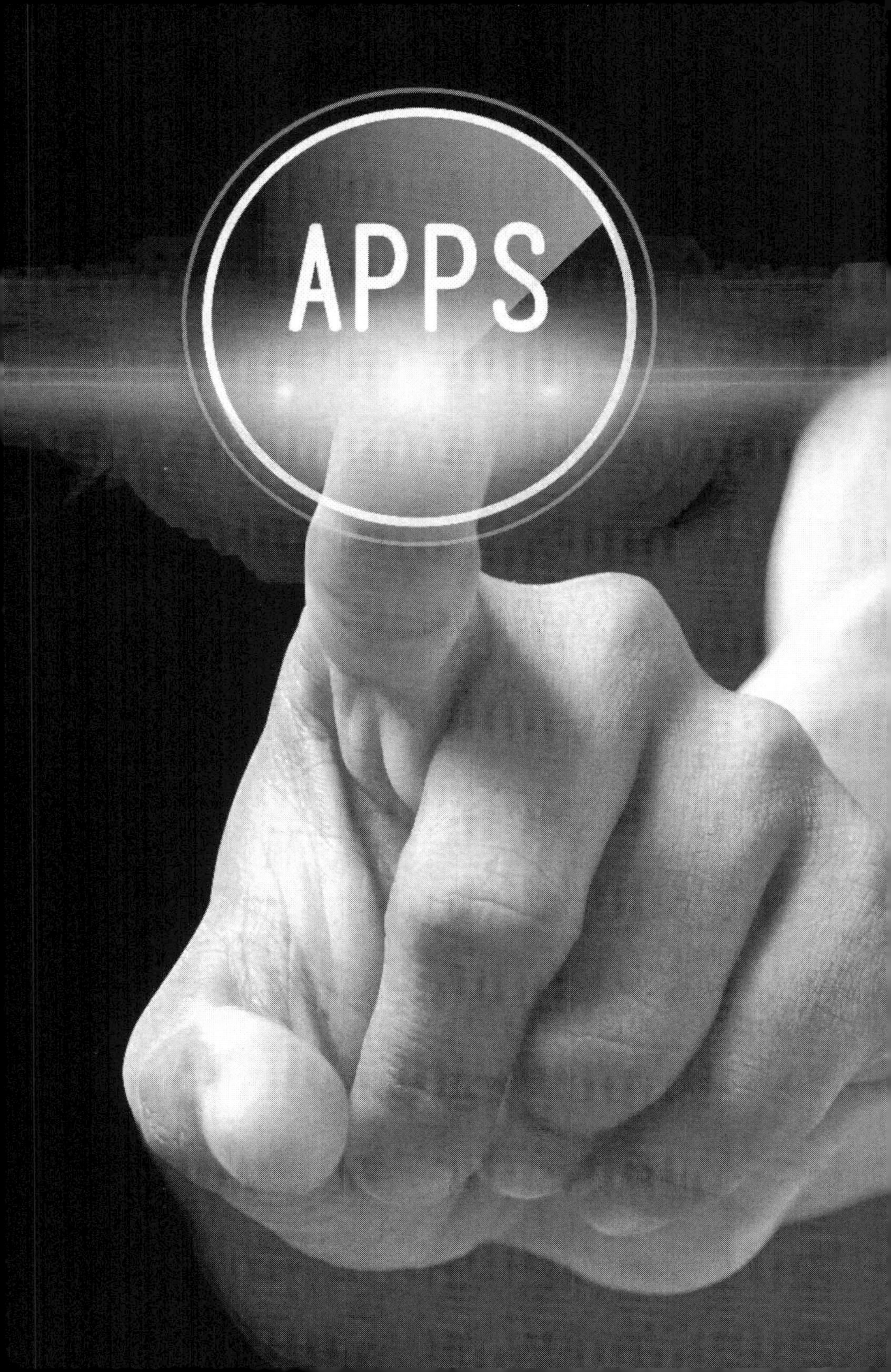
APPS

## ALARM

If your parent needs to take medication every four hours like our mom did, it might be a good idea to set an alarm so you don't forget and also to write down when the medicine is taken.

## ALKALINE

A phrase we heard early and often is "Cancer can't grow in an alkaline environment." We found a list of alkaline foods and helped our mom select foods that were more alkaline than acidic when possible.

She bought a couple of books on the subject including "The Acid Alkaline Food Guide: A Quick Reference to Foods & Their Effect on pH Levels," by Dr. Susan E. Brown and Larry Trivieri, Jr.

She also tested her pH level and drank ginger water throughout the day to make her body more alkaline.

## AMERICAN CANCER SOCIETY

The American Cancer Society is an organization that offers services to help cancer patients and their families manage life with cancer. Its website and programs provide information ranging from going through treatment and recovery, to finding emotional support. The American Cancer Society has many local offices across the country and provides free wigs and makeup for cancer patients. www.cancer.org

# APPS

Apps can help patients track cancer treatments. Although depending upon your parent, he or she might prefer paper and pen. But if you are going to be around your parent a lot, you can keep track of everything for him or her on an app instead.

We weren't aware of these apps when our mom was diagnosed so we haven't really checked them out, but we heard about them and thought we would pass along the information. We're sure there are other cancer apps in development at this time as there are tons of details to keep track of during cancer treatment.

Here are five free apps that are available in the iTunes App Store and Google Play.

1. Cancer Net: Developed by the American Society of Clinical Oncology. It has guides to 120 types of cancer with sample questions to ask a physician. There is a symptom tracker and you can save info about prescriptions including photos of labels and bottles.

2. Pocket Cancer Care Guide: Developed by the National Coalition for Cancer Survivorship. It has a glossary of medical terminology, links appointments to a calendar and you can record answers from doctors and nurses.

3. Create to Heal: Developed by the Women Wings Create to Heal TM program. This app helps relieve stress during treatment and recovery by using the healing power of creativity. You can play music and use art, color, meditation and creative writing tools.

4. My PearlPoint Cancer Side Effects Helper: Developed by PearlPoint Cancer Support. This app helps users cope with side effects by understanding why the body is reacting in a certain way. It has tools for improving day-to-day living.

5. Chemo Brain Doc Notes FREE: Developed by a cancer patient and the CrowdCare Foundation, Inc. Cancer treatment can lead to thinking and memory problems. This app helps patients manage treatment information. It has a feature to record and play back doctor visits.

# B

Benign

Biopsy

Brighten (The Home)

Books

## BENIGN

A tumor that is not cancerous.

## BIOPSY

A small sample of tissue taken from the body to examine it more closely. A biopsy can confirm that a tumor is cancerous.

## BRIGHTEN (THE HOME)

Does a dark, gloomy, depressing home sound appealing to a sick patient? No! Even though the doctors can give medicine and prescribe things to physically heal, home should be a calming and relaxing place to be.

When our mom was diagnosed, we brightened our house. Jacqueline used a yellow stencil on a living room wall and we made everything more cheerful and colorful! It brightened our mom's spirits and everyone who came into the living room.

## BOOKS

We reviewed about 60 books on cancer when our mom was diagnosed. We bought out all the relevant books at the local Barnes & Noble, although there was not a very big selection at our local bookstore. We checked out books at the local library, including books that could be ordered from neighboring branch libraries online. We also found many used books online for only a penny (plus shipping).

While a lot of information is available on the Internet, your parent might prefer a book and you can help your parent find books on his or her particular cancer. It is sometimes easier to refer to a book that your parent can underline or make notes in, or use a Post-it® Note, than to try to find the website again, especially if your parent is spending a lot of time resting.

Below are some of our mom's favorite books.

1. "Crazy Sexy Cancer Tips," by Kris Carr (A fun book with lots of practical tips. Note: Kris Carr is no relation to us.)

2. "Radical Remission: Surviving Cancer Against All Odds," by Kelly A. Turner PhD. (A book that offers hope and alternate treatments when it looks hopeless.)

3. "The Acid Alkaline Food Guide - A Quick Reference to Foods & Their Effect on pH Levels," by Dr. Susan E. Brown and Larry Trivieri, Jr. (A list of foods that are alkaline.)

4. "Chemo Companion Pocket Guide - Tips and Wisdom to Prepare for Your Chemo Journey," by Jean E. Sprengel, M.D. (A fun colorful book free from our mom's doctor, published by Merck, and currently available used online.)

5. "Foods that Harm and Foods that Heal: The Best and Worst Choices to Treat your Ailments Naturally," by the Editors of Reader's Digest. (Colorful photos and packed with details.)

6. "100 Questions & Answers about Esophageal Cancer, Second Edition," by Pamela K. Ginex and Maureen Jingeleski. Our mom bought an extra copy for our grandma so she could also understand the disease and treatments.

The "100 Question & Answers" series are excellent, concise books. They focus on one particular cancer and there are about 20 or so book titles available.

Below are the titles we saw available online in this series. If they are anything like "100 Questions & Answers about Esophageal Cancer," the layout should be clear, they should be easy to read, and provide encouragement and suggestions.

The "100 Questions & Answers" series is published by Jones and Barlett Learning and includes titles about the following cancers: advanced and metastatic breast, bladder, biliary, breast, cervical, colorectal, gastric, leukemia, liver, lung, lymphoma, kidney, myeloma, ovarian, pancreatic, prostate cancer, triple negative breast cancer and uterine.

www.jblearning.com

# C

Cancer Compass

CaringBridge

Case Manager

Chemo Brain & Chemo Curls

Chemotherapy

Clinical Trials

Cold

College

Complications

CT Scan

Cure Magazine

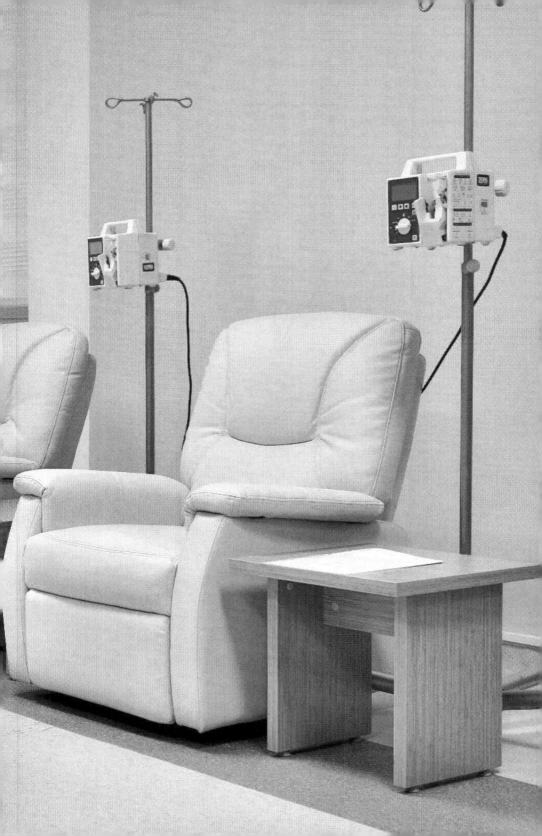

# CANCER

Cancer is a condition in which cells in the body start to grow abnormally and begin to harm the person. This leads to a tumor.

# CANCER COMPASS

This website cancercompass.com is one of many forums for people who want to share their experiences with a specific type of cancer, exchange ideas and provide support to patients or caregivers.

Our mom found it very helpful as she connected with people who had the specific side effect she was suffering from after surgery and she found their suggestions useful.

Here is a list of the message boards for specific types of cancer on Cancer Compass: bladder, bone, breast cancer, colon, esophageal, gynecological, kidney, leukemia, liver, lung, melanoma, pancreatic, prostate, stomach cancer and testicular.

In addition to the message boards for specific cancers, Cancer Compass has message boards for topics that can apply to most cancers:
After Treatment: Emotional Support, Nutritional Concerns, Side Effects
Diagnosis: Diagnostic Imaging, Lab Tests, Other Tests
Nutrition: Diet, Recipes, Supplements
Prevention: Genetics, Prevention Tips, Screening
Treatments: Alternative Treatments, Clinical Trials & Research, Conventional Treatments, Insurance Questions, Spiritual
Caregivers: Lifestyle, Support, Tips, Bereavement

# CARINGBRIDGE

If you want to keep your friends and family updated on your parent's medical condition, one easy way is through a free CaringBridge online account. www.caringbridge.org

According to the website, "Since 1997, more than half a million CaringBridge websites have been created. One in nine people in the U.S. have used CaringBridge to rally support for a loved one during a health journey, and our reach extends to 236 countries and territories around the world."

You can let people who sign up for updates hear when your parent is having chemotherapy, radiation or surgery and give updates you want to share, and they can offer encouragement and support through this website. You can keep your privacy by selecting who can have access to your account.

We didn't use CaringBridge ourselves, but it is helpful to people who have a lot of friends or family they want to update and we have kept up to date on the conditions of our friends through CaringBridge over the years.

# CASE MANAGER

After your parent is diagnosed with cancer, he or she will probably be assigned a case manager. The role of the case manager is to coordinate all of the cancer treatments the doctor has ordered, as well as to advocate on your parent's behalf.

## CHEMO BRAIN & CHEMO CURLS

According to the Mayo Clinic, chemo brain is a common term used by cancer survivors to describe thinking and memory problems that can occur after cancer treatment. Chemo brain is also called chemo fog, cognitive dysfunction or chemotherapy-related cognitive impairment.

If your parent is having chemo, you might need to step up your game in terms of keeping an eye on the finances or other tasks your parent handled before. For example, we were having some house repairs done by a handyman when our mom was having chemo, and she was in such a blur she couldn't even figure out how much to pay him and almost paid him double. Fortunately, we were there to keep an eye on what was happening and what she had agreed to pay for.

After chemotherapy is over and hair starts to grow back, the texture and color might be different from the original hair. If it is very curly—and that's a new look for your parent—it is called "chemo curls." We're not sure how long it lasts, but two years later our mom still has chemo curls! She's able to straighten her hair, or she can go for the bouncy, curly look.

## CHEMOTHERAPY

There are many types of chemotherapy drugs and we'll explain how you can help your parent during chemotherapy.

Chemotherapy is a drug that is usually given to a cancer patient through either an IV (intravenous) line through their arm or possibly a PICC line, which is a tube inserted near their shoulder that stays in place for possibly many weeks and provides a slow administration of the drug.

Chemo is usually done in a hospital or clinic and your parent will sit in a chair and be attached to IV equipment for many hours. Your job, if you are accompanying your parent, is to keep his or her spirits up, provide the food and drink that you packed, and otherwise comfort or entertain your parent. We were fortunate to be given a blanket by the hospital staff that was handmade and donated for patients. It can get very cold in the chemo infusion rooms, so be prepared.

The chemotherapy itself doesn't hurt any more than an IV, but it takes a long time. Our mom's chemo took about six hours. Your parent will probably feel a little strange when all the chemicals are in his or her body.

There are some arrangements you'll want to make ahead of time. You'll need a licensed driver to take your parent home. Also, you will need to have filled the prescriptions to treat the chemo-therapy side effects so you can give your parent the medication the doctor ordered.

In our mother's case, her doctor prescribed a lot of anti-nausea medication. Her doctor suggested taking the medication before the nausea hits. We set up a spreadsheet with details of when to take the pills and made sure she took them, because she could fall asleep or not focus on when she needed to take the medication or if she had already taken it.

# CLINICAL TRIALS

Clinical trials are research studies that test if a new medical approach works in people. You can ask your parent's oncologist about possible clinical trials or search for them on the Internet. Some sites that list clinical trials include:

National Institutes of Health
www.nih.gov/health-information/nih-clinical-research-trials-you/basics

National Heart, Lung and Blood Institute
www.nhlbi.nih.gov/studies/clinicaltrials/

American Cancer Society
www.cancer.org/treatment/treatmentsandsideeffects/clinicaltrials/app/clinical-trials-matching-service.aspx

National Cancer Institute
www.cancer.gov/about-cancer/treatment/clinical-trials/search

We checked out clinical trials in the beginning right after our mom's diagnosis and wrote to one organization but never heard back. We were confident that the traditional treatment for her disease was a safe first approach so we didn't feel it was necessary to pursue clinical trials.


# COLD

If your parent has chemotherapy or loses a lot of weight from treatment, he or she might be more susceptible to being cold. It might be a good time to stock up on some sweaters and blankets. Our mom usually had a heating pad on her lap.

# COMPLICATIONS

For cancer treatments such as chemotherapy, radiation and surgery, the physician or nurse will most likely provide your parent with a list of possible complications and what to do about them. Although this list will sound overwhelming and scary, it's good to keep it handy so you know what to do if your parent develops one of the symptoms.

We communicated with the physicians by email and phone. We also had a 24-hour nurse hotline we could call, and the ER was only about 15 minutes away. Be sure you know who to contact if there are complications and how to contact someone during non-business hours.

# CT SCAN

CT is also known as a CAT (Computerized Axial Tomography) scan. It is a diagnostic procedure that combines an x-ray with a computer and creates pictures with a three-dimensional quality. An IV dye is usually injected in the vein which creates a contrast for improved imaging. Sometimes oral contrast is used as well.

The patient lies still on a table and the scanner moves around the patient's body. It doesn't hurt except for the IV. CT scans can be used for cancer diagnosis or to determine if the cancer has spread or returned.

## CURE MAGAZINE

*Cure Magazine* is a free quarterly magazine for cancer patients, survivors and caregivers. The subscription comes with an annual cancer guide. The website also provides information about cancer news and events. www.curetoday.com

# D

DECORATING
(THE HOSPITAL ROOM)

DEEP VEIN THROMBOSIS (DVT)

DENTIST

DESIGNER BARF BAG

DISABILITY

DISABLED PARKING PERMIT

DOCTORS

DRIVING

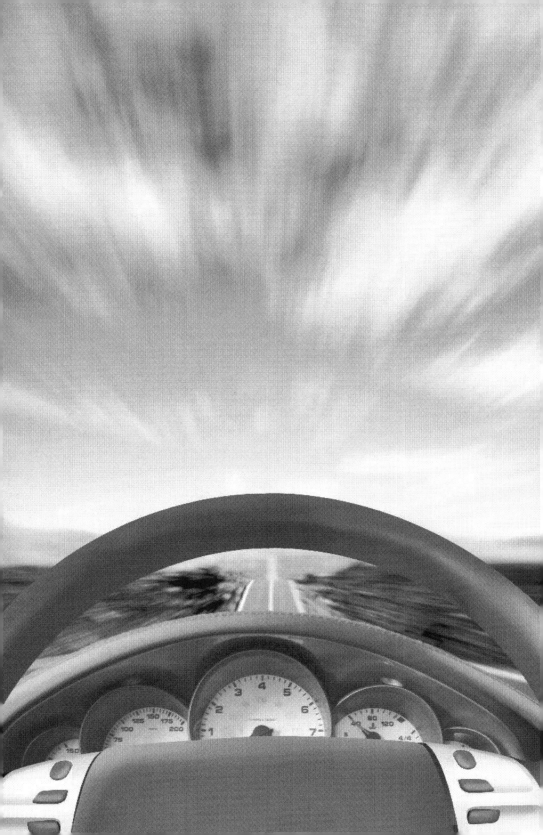

# DECORATING (THE HOSPITAL ROOM)

Being in a hospital room, whether it's for a few hours or a few days, can often feel like a sterile, white and cold environment. To bring some life and happiness to the room, try hanging a few uplifting signs or colorful decorations.

To decorate the hospital room that would be our mom's living quarters for the ten days after her surgery, we made a huge poster that said, "We love you Mommy" and "You are strong" written in colorful marker. It also had drawings of yellow and blue hearts, along with pictures of our family and pets. It was a nice pick-me-up for both our mom and us—as well as for the hospital staff—to look at every day in the hospital.

# DEEP VEIN THROMBOSIS (DVT)

A DVT is a blood clot in a deep vein. Look out for this complication from chemotherapy. Here is a link for more info from the U.S. Department of Health and Human Services. www.nhlbi.nih.gov/health/health-topics/topics/dvt

Our mom had a DVT and a pulmonary embolism from chemotherapy. Fortunately, there is treatment but it is best to catch it early. In the hospital with the DVT and pulmonary embolism, our mom was on an IV for blood clots. She also had to give herself two injections of Lovenox daily for six months. Although a pill version of a blood thinner like Coumadin (Warfarin) is used by some people, her doctor told her because she was being treated for cancer she needed Lovenox.

## DENTIST

A trip to the dentist is a good idea before cancer treatment, because sometimes there are limitations on what dental procedures can be performed on someone receiving cancer treatment.

## DESIGNER BARF BAGS

We read about designer barf bags in "Crazy Sexy Cancer Tips." We thought it would make the chemo experience a little more fun. Although we bought some of the purple bags with designs our mom took the prescribed amount of anti-nausea medication and never needed the bags. Large selections of these items are available on web sites such as www.barfboutique.com.

## DISABILITY

You can help your parent review the requirements for private disability and disability through the federal government for Social Security Disability (SSD) and Supplemental Security Income (SSI) or state disability programs that might be available because of your parent's cancer diagnosis and condition.

## DISABLED PARKING PERMIT

If your parent needs a disabled parking permit, you can usually get the form off the Internet from your state's Department of Motor Vehicles.

You will then need to get your parent's doctor to sign the form. You can get a temporary disabled parking permit from your state's Department of Motor Vehicles or the Auto Club.

## DOCTORS

It's often good to get a second opinion for treatment. You might find that you are rushed into a chemotherapy and radiation schedule, but hopefully you can have time to get a second opinion from surgeons.

## DRIVING

Your parent probably won't be able to drive for a while after a surgery. Some medications should not be taken before driving. Also, depending on the extent of your parent's surgery, he or she might find it very uncomfortable to drive. To overcome this, our mom put a bed pillow behind her and another in front of her and then put her seat belt over the pillow. This made it more comfortable for her to drive. If you don't drive, you might be able to find a friend or neighbor who can help, or you can use Uber, www.uber.com, a taxi, or other driving service.

# E

EMERGENCY ROOM (ER)

ENCOURAGEMENT

ENERGY

ESOPHAGEAL CANCER SYMPTOMS

EXERCISE

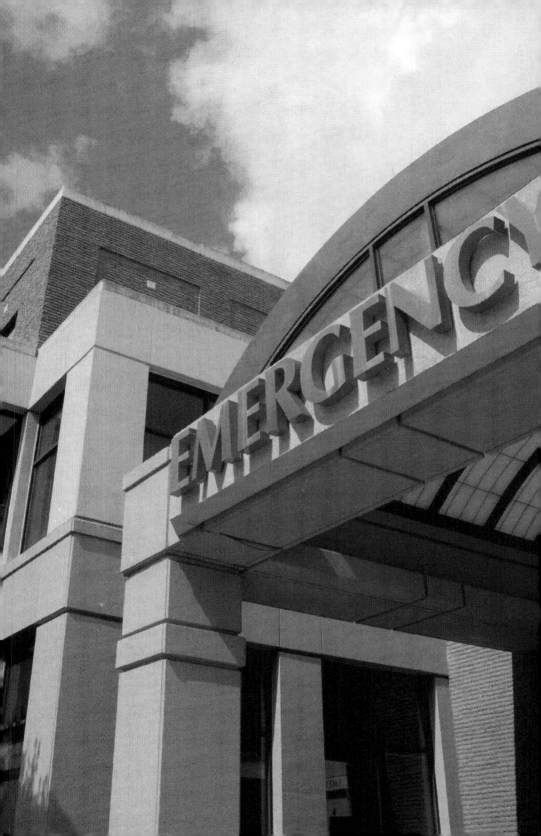

# EMERGENCY ROOM (ER)

If your doctor or the nurse hotline suggests your parent go to the emergency room, or he or she is suffering from some of the possible side effects of treatment that requires emergency care, you might want to bring yourself some food, something to read, something to write on and some warm clothes. It could be a long visit!

Be sure to bring the cell phone and charger, too. We had many long nights and early morning visits to the ER. On the positive side, there's never much traffic driving home at 3 a.m.!

# ENCOURAGEMENT

There were days when our mom didn't want to do anything or eat anything and was overall in a depressed mood. We tried to combat that attitude with words of encouragement by listing out everything for which we were grateful.

When she ate a little bite of something—that was a lot for her considering all the effects of chemotherapy and radiation she was dealing with—we cheered her on and always asked, in the sweetest voice, "Would you like another bite?"

Repetition is important and helped keep our mom on the right track. Just a little encouragement can go a long way! We managed to get our mom to eat a little bit more with just a little en-couragement.

## ENERGY

Helping a parent with cancer can be very tiring. Whether you're accompanying him or her to doctor's appointments, providing care after surgery, getting food or going for a walk together, it's very likely you will run out of energy. While there is no perfect way to regain energy, one important method is sleep.

While we were helping our mom, we always tried to go to bed at a reasonable hour and make sure we got enough sleep. This makes you less groggy or irritable and fit to take on whatever your parent needs help with the next day. Depending on what your parent is going through, you might need to get up several times in the night to help. So it is best to savor the sleep whenever you can get it.

## ESOPHAGEAL CANCER SYMPTOMS

You can get an overview of esophageal cancer or any type of cancer from www.cancer.net.

The people we told about our mother's condition asked how she found out that she had cancer and what symptoms she had. Our mom had trouble swallowing and would choke on food occasionally.

Below, from the cancer.net website, are the symptoms of esophageal cancer, which is a cancer that is sometimes difficult to detect.

"The esophagus is a 10-inch long, hollow, muscular tube that connects the throat to the stomach. It is part of a person's gastrointestinal (GI) tract. When a person swallows, the walls of the esophagus squeeze together to push food down into the stomach.

"People with esophageal cancer may experience the following symptoms or signs. Sometimes, people with esophageal cancer do not show any of these symptoms. Or, these symptoms may be caused by a medical condition that is not cancer.

- Difficulty and pain with swallowing, particularly when eating meat, bread, or raw vegetables. As the tumor grows, it can block the pathway to the stomach. Even liquid may be painful to swallow.
- Pressure or burning in the chest
- Indigestion or heartburn
- Vomiting
- Frequent choking on food
- Unexplained weight loss
- Coughing or hoarseness
- Pain behind the breastbone or in the throat"

Source: www.cancer.net

If your parent ever gets these symptoms, it is a good idea for him or her to be checked for esophageal cancer.


## EXERCISE

Doctors will often suggest some exercise to patients even during treatment for cancer. But when a parent is having chemotherapy, it's sometimes not a good idea to be around other people without wearing a face mask due to the risk of infection. It's therefore might not be a good idea to go to a gym.

To make it easier for our mom to get some exercise, we got a small stationary bike and some small weights at home.

# F

FACE MASK

FEEDING TUBE

FENDING
(FOR ONESELF)

FINANCES

FOOD

FRIENDS & FAMILY

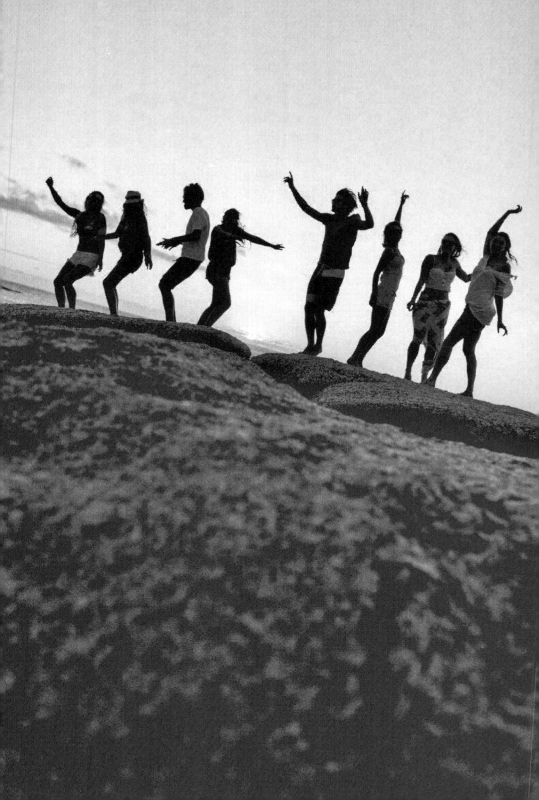

# FACE MASK

Your parent's oncologist might recommend that your parent wear a face mask during certain days or weeks of the chemotherapy when susceptibility to infection is the greatest. The masks are the small ones that cover the mouth and nose and strap around the ears. We got some from our mother's doctor, but they are also available at most pharmacies or online.

# FEEDING TUBE

We're not sure how common this is after cancer surgery, but our mom had a feeding tube while she was in the hospital and for two weeks after she came home.

The feeding tube was surgically implanted into her belly wall to her small intestine during the surgery to remove her esophagus. It was sewn to her abdomen and taped down. It was connected by a valve to the feeding tube apparatus that was about five feet high and on wheels and was kept near her bed and plugged in so it could operate properly.

We didn't know anything about feeding tubes in the beginning and thought that the feeding tube would go down her nose or mouth.

When she wasn't connected to the feeding tube apparatus that held the food, the part that protruded from her mid-section was not very big. It was hard to notice if she wore a sweater or baggy clothes to cover it.

Because our mom was physically very weak and her mind wasn't working too well because of the narcotic medications, we set up the feeding tube machine for her, hung the liquid food, connected it to the apparatus and set the computer dials so it would be regulated properly.

She had the feeding tube on all night for the first two weeks after she came home.

We could also use the feeding tube to give her medication because she couldn't swallow pills. We crushed the pills and diluted them with slightly warm water. It's kind of weird but our mom said she could feel the liquid going into her small intestine if it was too cold or too hot.

Just like Goldilocks trying out the three bears' porridge, our mom would feel the water with her finger to make sure it was just the right temperature before she would let us stick it in the syringe so she would get it into her feeding tube.

We had to flush the tube, or clean it before and after every feeding or delivering anything into the tube to prevent it from clogging.

Commercially prepared feeding tube products are available and probably covered by your insurance. We read that some people who wanted organic or vegan foods, or had specific preferences, made their own food for the feeding tube. We didn't do this.

Our mom really didn't like the feeding tube and she worked very hard to be able to eat food by mouth so she could wean off the feeding tube. She was thrilled when the doctor agreed to remove the feeding tube after only two weeks, because some esophageal cancer patients remain on the feeding tube for many months.

Feeding tube machines may seem overwhelming at first but are actually very user friendly and after a few tries the nurse was even calling us pros!

## FENDING (FOR ONESELF)

When a parent is sick and no longer able to provide the level of care that he or she provided to you before the illness, you might have to buy your own groceries and cook and graciously accept food from friends.

You might also find you have to do a lot more around the house than you did before your parent got cancer.

## FINANCES

You might take over some of the bill paying responsibilities from your parent, or at least learn how to log in to their online banking account in case of an emergency, if he or she needs help. If finances are tight because your parent can't work for health reasons, you can help your parent check out what other sources of income might be available through the government or elsewhere.

If you need money to help pay medical insurance co-pays, you can check out gofundme.com or other fundraising websites.

Many community support groups help those undergoing cancer treatment to raise funds to support a family. Your friends and family might have suggestions or connections to help with the bill paying during this time.

Some organizations that provide financial support for cancer patients or provide air travel expenses and hotels for those supporting family and friends with cancer are listed below:

American Cancer Society, Hope Lodge and Extended Stay America

www.cancer.org/treatment/supportprogramsservices/patientlodging/index

Joe's House

www.joeshouse.org

Freebies and Discounts for Cancer Patients

www.1uponcancer.com/freebies-and-discounts-for-cancer-patients/

Cancer.net

www.cancer.net/navigating-cancer-care/financial-considerations/financial-resources

## FOOD

Going from a set meal plan by nurses and doctors after surgery, to whatever is in your home fridge, your parent will need help finding what to eat and being able to eat it.

This was especially true for our mom after her surgery that removed her esophagus and half her stomach. She had very restricted food issues and could have serious consequences if she ate the wrong thing or too much at one time.

Whatever food your parent wants, it might be helpful to write it down and keep track of it in the beginning until your parent is up to getting his or her own food again.

## FUN

In the midst of cancer and all of the doom and gloom associated with it, it's important to try and have fun. While it may be hard at first to force fun into the mix, it's definitely possible and can really change the mood around.

We would have fun braiding our mom's hair in the hospital or pretending the wet sponge on a stick we gave our mom to moisten her tongue was a Popsicle or lollipop.

The nursing staff can also sometimes add to the fun. One of the nurses would make a heart on our mom's bed out of baby powder. Those little touches can really make all the difference.

During our mom's chemo, radiation and surgery we didn't have much time to get out but we occasionally went shopping and went to Disneyland once with her in a wheelchair after the pulmonary embolism when she could barely walk.

## FRIENDS & FAMILY

The significant people in your life can help you through the cancer process. Cancer patients will have different opinions about sharing the news and details about the disease.

In our family, we were very busy dealing with the cancer right after the diagnosis and we weren't ready to share the news with lots of people except a couple of our mom's close friends.

Later we shared the news with others. Our friends proved to be a big help both at the hospital and at home. Talk with your parent about who he or she feels comfortable telling and how much your parent wants to share with your friends and family.

# G

GENETICS

GINGER

GLASSES

GROCERIES DELIVERED

GUARDIAN

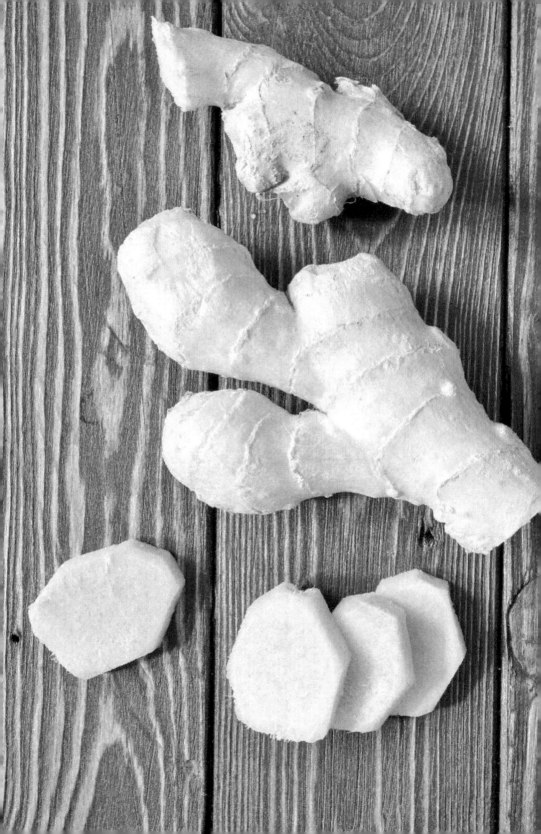

## GENETICS

It is natural to wonder if your parent has the type of cancer that you might get yourself one day. It might be worth doing some research to see if there is a genetic link, if you should be tested for a specific gene, or if you should be on the lookout for symptoms in the future. The American Cancer Society provides some background information on this topic.

http://www.cancer.org/cancer/cancercauses/geneticsandcanc er/heredity-and-cancer

Our mom was concerned that we might have a predisposition to getting a certain type of cancer, so she met with a genetics counselor who reviewed our family tree and all the different types of cancers our ancestors had, to the extent that our mom had the information.

## GINGER

Ginger is a highly alkaline-forming food. Every morning our mother would peel and chop up a small piece of ginger, about 3/4 of an inch long and boil it with lots of water for about 10 minutes. She would then strain it and drink it warm throughout the day.

She got this tip from a man who had survived 18 years with esophageal cancer and he based much of it on the Ayurvedic remedies from India. Lemon water can also be used to make the body more alkaline — which has been said to prevent cancer growth.

## GLASSES

If your parent is having surgery and wears contact lenses, you might want to make sure he or she also has glasses to bring to the hospital. It's a good time to make sure the prescription is current or possibly get an updated pair.

## GROCERIES DELIVERED

If you don't live within walking distance of grocery stores or can't get to a store, a lot of grocery stores now deliver groceries with a reasonable delivery charge. Some companies charges a flat fee for unlimited grocery delivery per year.

## GUARDIAN

This is our least favorite part out of all of this. Guardians. It's just too weird, too unbearably sad to think about. But you have to get through it. One day our mom sat us down and we talked about who would take care of us if our mom wasn't there.

If you or your siblings are under 18 and you don't have another parent, you will want to make sure your parent has made plans for a guardian—someone who will be legally responsible for you if your parent is not alive.

Your parent can have a legal document prepared that selects a guardian. It is a good idea to have clear communication with the potential guardian to make sure they are available and they see eye-to-eye with your parent regarding how you should be raised, where you would live and finances.

Our mom talked to our potential guardian and we were aware of all the details and felt it was a good plan.

Remember that all of this is precautionary. We hope that you will never need any of this—legal documents about wills, trusts and guardians—but it will put your and your parent's mind at rest, as we know it did for us. Once you're done writing and checking all this stuff, you can get on with your life and enjoy your time with your parent!

# H

HAIR

HOME HEALTH CARE

HOMEWORK

HOPE

HOSPICE

HOSPITAL GOWNS

HOSPITAL RANKINGS
(*U.S. NEWS & WORLD REPORT*)

HYPNOTHERAPY

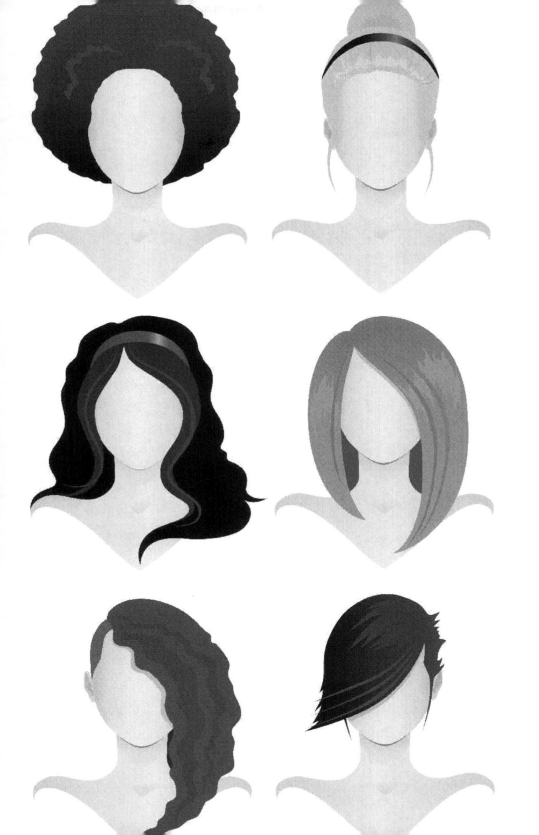

# HAIR

Where to start?

Hair loss can be one of the most visible signs of cancer. Each patient has his or her own approach to dealing with the challenge, from shaving off all the hair to buying an expensive human-hair wig. If the head is shaved, or the hair starts thinning on top, beanies or hats are good ways to stay warm and cover up the changes in hair thickness.

# HOME HEALTH CARE

You and your parent should check to see what home health care his or her insurance would cover. Home health care is a medically trained person coming to your house to take care of your parent.

If your parent's insurance doesn't cover home health care, there are outside organizations that can be used.

# HOMEWORK

Life and death situations seem so much more important than tedious homework. And they are, but if you're a student, homework still needs to get done. Talk with your teachers about your family situation if you feel you may not be doing your best while your parent is being treated or if you want them to know why you are more tired, sad or stressed out.

Teachers can be very understanding and while they may not give you accommodations, they will be aware of your situation.

# HOPE

A cancer diagnosis is a terrible thing to hear, and it may be easy to lose all hope, but you shouldn't. No matter how bad the situation may seem, there is always a reason to hope the situation will get better and then work toward a positive result.

When we found our mom had a rare and deadly cancer, we initially wanted to just curl up in a ball and lose all hope. Instead, we stood tall and remained hopeful to fight the cancer. Two years later the hope has paid off thus far and our mom is doing so much better.

# HOSPICE

Our goal was to be optimistic during the cancer process, but it's also important to be realistic and as such, somewhat detached from the actual situation. Depending on the type and stage of your parent's cancer, you might want to look into hospice care. Hospice is a place your parent can stay if he or she is terminally ill. You can also have hospice care come to your home. While this can be sad to think about, just go through the steps logically and always remain positive and loving toward your parent.

# HOSPITAL GOWNS

If your parent wants a more fashionable hospital gown than the one provided at the hospital, we found that they are available online.

We got colorful gowns with interesting designs that were also suitable for hospital use because they had snaps at the top so that doctors or nurses could attach tubes. The colorful gowns brightened our mom's day. One company we liked was Gownies. www.gownies.com

Later our grandma wore the gowns when she was in the hospital and she paraded up and down the hall modeling them for the other patients and nurses!

## HOSPITAL RANKINGS (*U.S. NEWS & WORLD REPORT*)

*U.S. News & World Report* has a ranking of the top cancer hospitals in the U.S. You can also do a search by type of cancer and location.

www.health.usnews.com/best-hospitals/rankings/cancer

## HYPNOTHERAPY

Preparing for a surgery, especially a high-risk surgery, requires preparation on all levels. Getting the subconscious mind ready to get the best results possible can be accomplished through hypno-therapy — at least that is what our mom did.

Our mom asked her surgeon for the name of a patient who was willing to discuss what worked for her before and after the surgery. The main thing the patient recommended was hypno-therapy, and she gave our mother the name and contact infor-mation for the hypnotherapist.

Our mom had never done anything like this before but was willing to try anything and everything to have a successful outcome.

With two phone sessions lasting about an hour or so each, our mom got a personalized one-hour CD that she could listen to in order to prepare her subconscious mind for the surgery.

It seemed to work! Our mom was very calm going into the surgery and said the exact phrase after the surgery that she told the hypnotherapist she would say after the surgery. "Yeah! We did it!"

The hypnotherapist helped our mom visualize what the surgeon would say after the surgery — namely that "it was very successful, even better than expected!" After the operation, the surgeon said the results were "phenomenal." Having a positive attitude going into the surgery really made us all more relaxed.

Our mom used Cynthia McDonald, Ph.D., Certified Clinical and Medical Hypnotherapist, Transformative Living, LLC, 408 307-3183. Everything was done over the phone.

www.transformative-living.com

# I

INSURANCE

INTENSIVE CARE UNIT (ICU)

INTRAVENOUS (IV)

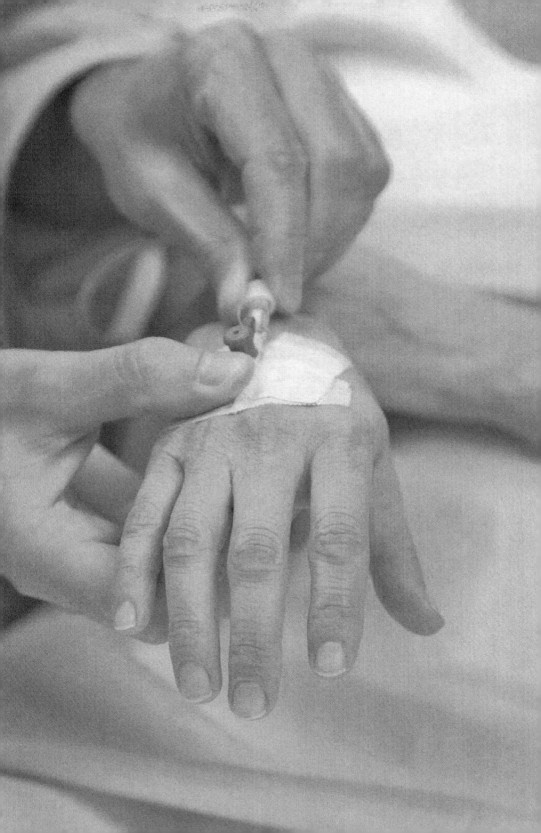

# INSURANCE

Cancer treatment is expensive. You can help your parent look into what aspects of the treatment—chemotherapy, radiation, surgery—your parent's insurance will cover. Your parent may already be aware of his or her coverage, but if not you can find a lot out by researching online or calling your parent's insurance plan or member services.

When you call, always write down who you talked with and what was said. This written record you keep can be used later if there are discrepancies in what was said.

You might need a separate file just for medical bills and receipts. It's also worth looking at the tax aspects of medical expenses.

If your parent's insurance plan doesn't pay for a service your parent feels is needed, you can look at out-of-plan options. If the service is not covered by your parent's insurance, your parent can request a referral. If the referral is denied, your parent can file a grievance, followed by an appeal and a possible appeal to the state governing board for insurance. The appeal to the state can be done on an emergency basis if your parent hasn't had the surgery or procedure yet, or can be filed after the fact and your parent has the chance of being reimbursed.

In California, when we were reviewing it, we read that about 60 percent of cases that are filed result in the patient getting what they requested, so it is worth pursuing.

We spent hours helping our mom navigate through the insurance restrictions and requirements and review the grievance and appeals process. We attached all the relevant medical documents and details because she wanted to go to the experienced surgeon with the best results, not the surgeon under her plan because patients treated under her plan died more frequently and had higher complication rates.

This was on top of everything else we needed to do while she was having chemotherapy and radiation, but we all felt that the best medical care we could find was necessary to have the best chances for success.

Your parent's medical services available through his or her insurance might be amazing and everything your parent needs, so you might not need to deal with this. However, just in case your parent wants options it's good to know where to get the forms, as well as the requirements and deadlines.

## INTENSIVE CARE UNIT (ICU)

This is the unit at a hospital that treats patients with severe and life threatening illnesses or injuries which require close moni-toring and special equipment. There is a higher staff-to-patient ratio and more advanced equipment and resources. Patients are transferred from one department at a hospital to the ICU if their condition worsens.

Our mom was in the ICU for seven days after her cancer surgery and then went to the regular ward, but her symptoms of a fast heartbeat (tachycardia) worsened, and so she was transferred back to the ICU.

If you are helping your parent in the ICU, you might be lucky enough to get a cot or chair to sleep on so you can spend the night. Some hospitals have family rooms that are down the hall.

If neither accommodation is available, the hospital might have an arrangement with a local hotel for a discounted rate if you are not near your home or if you don't have a family member or friend you can stay with. Some organizations also offer free hotel rooms for family who are visiting cancer patients in the hospital.

## INTRAVENOUS (IV)

IVs are used to regulate the flow rate of the drug into the blood stream. A nurse will insert a needle in the vein of the arm or hand, which can be painful for some people. Then it is taped down in place. For chemotherapy treatment, the nurse will connect the various containers with the chemo drugs that are on a stand next to the patient. The machines will beep and the nurse will check them regularly. The nurses we saw wore safety gowns and gloves in case the chemo container leaked, which can be harmful to those who don't need the drug.

One problem we noticed from all the IV's and blood draws that our mom had was that her veins were "blown" as a result of the cancer treatments. The nurses had a very difficult time getting needles in her and it caused a great deal of pain.

If you're with your parent, make a mental or written note as to which veins are good and which are bad and whether they roll which makes it difficult to get the needle in.

We learned the hard way to ask for the "sharp-shooter" or the person who is the most experienced at getting needles into challenging veins. We got in the habit of asking right off the bat for the supervisor who is the most skilled. It was sad to see someone stick our mom three times in different veins and still not be successful, then have the person who was the most skilled come in at the end and do it successfully.

# J

## JUGGLING
## (SCHOOLWORK & CAREGIVING)

## JUICING

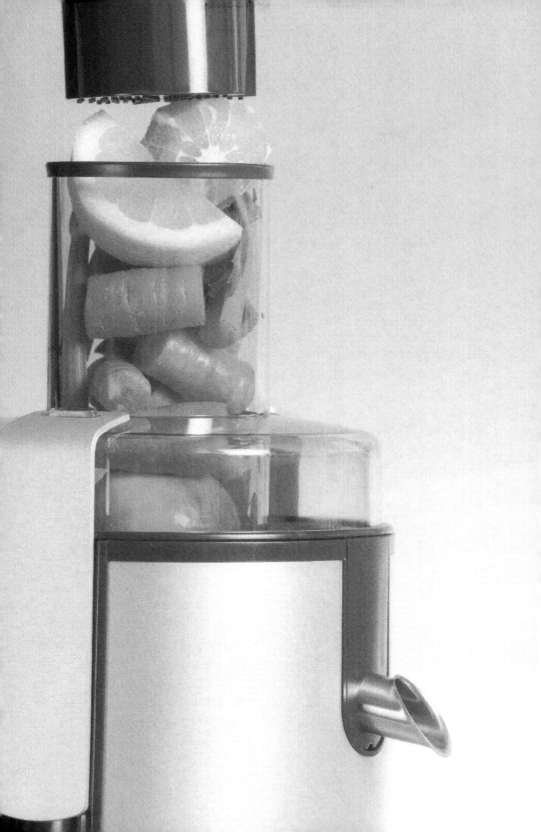

# JUGGLING (SCHOOLWORK & CAREGIVING)

A teenager's life can be very busy. High school or college, homework, sports, friends, and sleep? Now being punched in the face with a family member's illness can really jumble things up.

As a student and a caregiver to a parent, it is hard to get everything done. You might need to make some sacrifices on your extracurricular activities but it will be worth it in the long run.

Your teachers can probably work with you in terms of taking time off if you need to go to the hospital. Jacqueline was in 10th grade and took a week off from school with an independent contract program that allowed her to do the work at the hospital and turn in assignments and take tests when she returned.

If you can get a week or more off from school to take care of your parent in the hospital, through an independent contract, be sure to email, email, email.

Email your teachers and set up meetings with them to get all the assignments and material you will be missing. It's very important that you don't fall behind. Getting everything they say in an email will give you a hard copy of what they want you to accomplish in the time you are away.

Although she loves sports, Jacqueline chose not to pursue the volleyball team during her 10th grade year when our mom was having surgery, as it would take too much time. Katherine missed a few days during her first quarter at college to fly home to help her mother at the hospital after the surgery. She took a light course load her first quarter, didn't join any clubs or extracurricular activities, and didn't go to many social events.

Some colleges will allow students to take a leave of absence for a quarter, semester, year or longer so the student can help in a family medical situation or for other reasons. If you haven't started college but have been accepted, you might look into a gap year to delay the start of your freshman year.

## JUICING

You have probably read that juicing fresh organic vegetables, particularly kale, will go a long way in helping restore your parent's health. We read this in numerous books, including "Crazy Sexy Cancer Tips" by Kris Carr.

In addition to helping your parent select a juicer, buying and cutting up the vegetables, and cleaning the juicer is something your parent will probably really appreciate.

Juicing is a great way to get a lot of vitamins and minerals from fruits and vegetables all at once. Instead of having to eat food separately, your parent can just drink a juice and receive the same nutritional benefits.

Depending on what treatment your parent is having, he or she may not be able to eat very much or eat solid foods. Juicing can solve that problem. People usually juice raw fruits and vegetables. Raw is often the best form to consume these foods in because many foods lose some of their nutrients once cooked.

# K

KALE

KELOID SCAR

KIDS KONNECTED

KLEENEX®

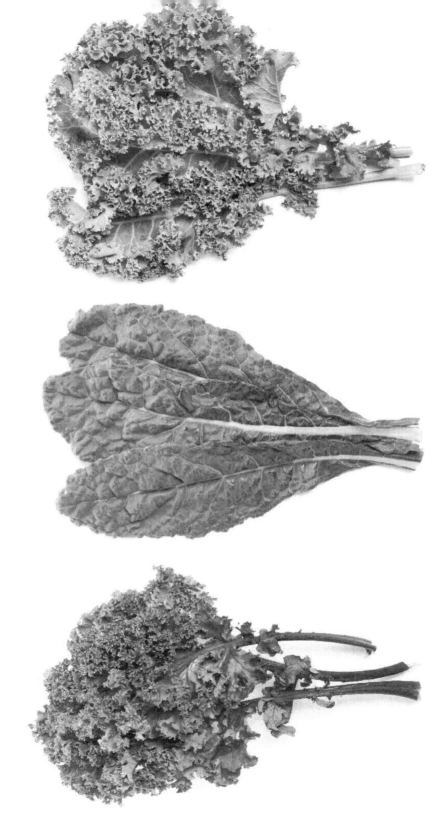

# KALE

Kale is known as a healthy vegetable. It has tons of nutrients, and in our quest to find the best foods for our mom to eat, kale was often at the top of the list. But, the one problem is our mom doesn't like kale, especially juiced.

There are ways to cook it to make it taste better. We tried baking it to make kale chips, but they still weren't a big hit. See if your parent likes or can tolerate kale. If regular kale doesn't strike his or her fancy, try baby kale. It's a less intense, less bitter flavor.

# KELOID SCAR

If your parent is planning to have surgery, you should be aware of how the scars may heal. One possibility is for your parent to have a keloid scar. This type of scar is raised, red, shiny, and extends beyond the borders of the original incision. Some people are more susceptible to keloid scars than others. Our mom didn't have keloid scars from her incisions but don't be alarmed if your parent's skin starts to form keloid scars after surgery.

Recent studies have shown that a tension off-loading device can result in an improved scar. www.embracescartherapy.com. You can also buy ointments and lotions to help the scar heal better. Although these ointments and lotions have not been scientifically proven, they are available from the pharmacy.

# KIDS KONNECTED

Kids Konnected is an organization whose mission is "to provide friendship, understanding, education and support for kids and teens who have a parent with cancer or have lost a parent with cancer." If you feel alone and would like to talk to others in your situation, Kids Konnected is a great resource. You can reach out on the following website: www.kidskonnected.org

## KLEENEX®

You never know when your parent will need a tissue, especially if he or she is in bed after surgery and can't get one without help. It's a good idea to always have Kleenex® or another type of tissue around the house or in the hospital just in case.

# L

LAUGHTER

THE LEAPFROG GROUP

LEMONS

LISTS

LYMPH NODES

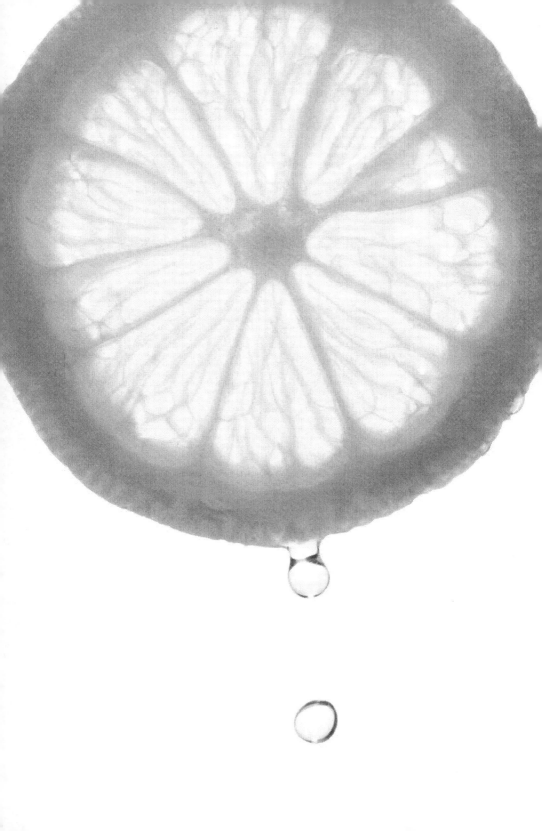

## LAUGHTER

Laughter is the best medicine, right? Well, actually it is.

Find little things like funny videos, DVDs or movies — they can really lighten your spirits. Laughter releases built-up stress and makes you happy again.

## THE LEAPFROG GROUP

If your parent is trying to select a hospital for treatment or surgery, this online guide to top hospitals might be helpful. It includes ratings for the success of our mom's high-risk surgery. It compares the statistical success for outcomes on a variety of factors for various hospitals.
www.leapfroggroup.org/patients.

## LEMONS

You wouldn't think that an acidic lemon would make your body more alkaline (basic), but it does. As you start to metabolize the lemon, your body's pH is actually raised, making it more basic. Therefore, lemons can be a good option to make your parent's body more alkaline.

## LISTS

While a parent is going through cancer treatment, there is a lot going on. From doctor's appointments to chemotherapy and radiation treatments and meal planning, there is a lot to keep track of.

We wanted to lighten the load for our mom and not have her feel too much of the burden of everything that there was to do. So we made lists.

We filled out a calendar with her doctor appointments and what we hoped to accomplish.

Together with her, we wrote a list of questions for each doctor and kept the notebook handy to jot down the answers as she spoke with each physician.

Once we were in the hospital after the surgery, we made a list of what our mom had to do each day, such as her breathing exercises (using an incentive spirometer) and walking and rinsing out her mouth, so she didn't have to try to remember or rely on the nurses to remind her.

## LYMPH NODES

Lymph nodes aren't body parts that a lot of people pay attention to. We don't remember learning much about them in high school biology class. But, they are very important in the realm of cancer.

The doctors will tell your parent if the cancer has spread to the lymph nodes, and it's not a good sign if it does.

Spreading means the cancer has metastasized and is traveling throughout the body. It is easier to treat cancer if it is localized (in one place), rather than if the tumor is metastasized and spread to other parts of the body.

The lymph nodes are part of the immune system and are found throughout the body. They are small, about one third of an inch, and are soft and round. Your body has between 500 and 700 lymph nodes.

Your parent's doctor may tell you that he or she plans to remove lymph nodes that are near the cancer during surgery. This is done as a precaution to make sure there is no cancer left in the body. Our mom had 77 lymph nodes around her esophagus removed during her surgery.

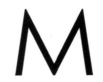

# M

MACHINES

MALIGNANCY

MASSAGE

MEDICATION

MEDITATION

METASTASIS

MRI

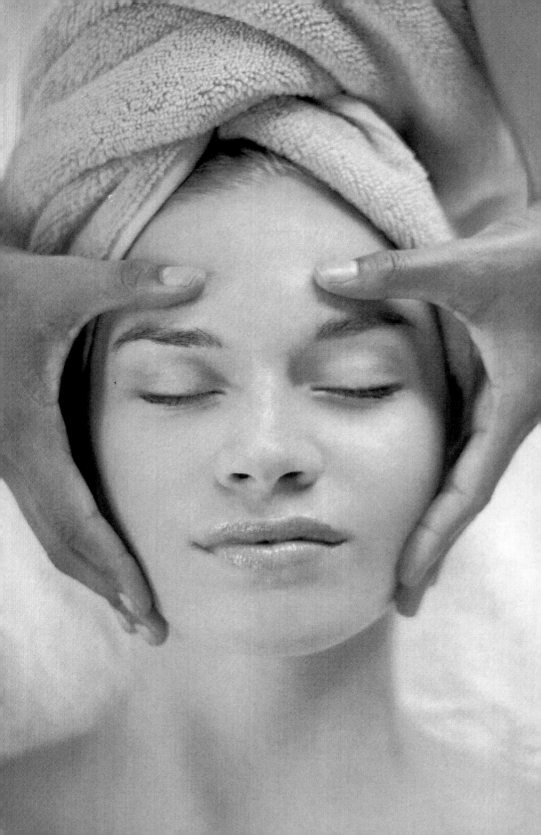

## MACHINES

There are many machines in a hospital room. Some beep, some are on wheels and some are connected to wires, cords, or sharp needles. While you probably won't be able to distinguish all the machines from one another, we tried our best to know what the most important ones were doing.

The blood pressure and heart monitor machine was always hooked up to our mom and we would check it to make sure her vitals were normal.

If we didn't know what a nurse was hooking her up to, we would always ask so that we, our mom, and the nurses were all on the same page with her treatment.

It's best to be proactive and understand the situation so you can help your parent if he or she needs anything or has questions.


## MALIGNANCY

Tumors that can grow and invade surrounding tissues and spread to other parts of the body are malignant. If a tumor is malignant that means it is cancerous.


## MASSAGE

Our mom's mentor who survived 18 years with esophageal cancer recommended daily self-massage as well as weekly massages at salons if possible.

The rationale for massages, according to our mom's mentor, is that it helps to work the toxins out of the body and stimulates the lymph nodes.

We did a little research on this and found mostly that massage was helpful in reducing stress.

www.cancercouncil.com.au/17958/b1000/massage-and-cancer-42/massage-and-cancer-benefits-of-touch/

Our mom enjoyed massages whenever possible during her treatments and she always looked and felt better after she returned from a massage. We found that there was a large range of prices and services for massages for almost every budget.


## MEDICATION

If your parent isn't able to swallow pills, you can buy a pill crusher, which is about the size of a lemon and costs about five dollars at a pharmacy or other store. There are also small devices that can cut a pill in half for you.

It's important to keep track of when medication is taken. If medication has to be taken around the clock, you can set an alarm. When our mom first came home from the hospital she had to take medication every four hours so we set alarms on our phones to ring at 3, 7 and 11 a.m. and p.m. It helped us to keep on track and saved us from missing a dose.

## MEDITATION

For many people, meditation is a great way to clear the mind and feel more stress free. This is a nice state of mind for anyone, especially someone going through a normally stressful time such as a cancer diagnosis and treatment. You can look for DVDs on meditation or watch YouTube videos on meditation with your parent. These videos could provide helpful tips to stay calm in stressful situations.

## METASTASIS

When the cancer has spread from the primary or original tumor to another part of the body it has metastasized.

## MRI (MAGNETIC RESONANCE IMAGING)

MRI stands for magnetic resonance imaging. It is an imaging tool used to look at various parts of the body, such as the brain, heart and abdomen. While our mother didn't need an MRI, this type of imaging can be used for diagnosis and staging of other types of cancers, including neurological cancer, prostate cancer and bone cancer.

# N

NAUSEA

NEIGHBORS

NEW NORMAL

NO EVIDENCE OF DISEASE (NED)

NOTEBOOKS

NURSES

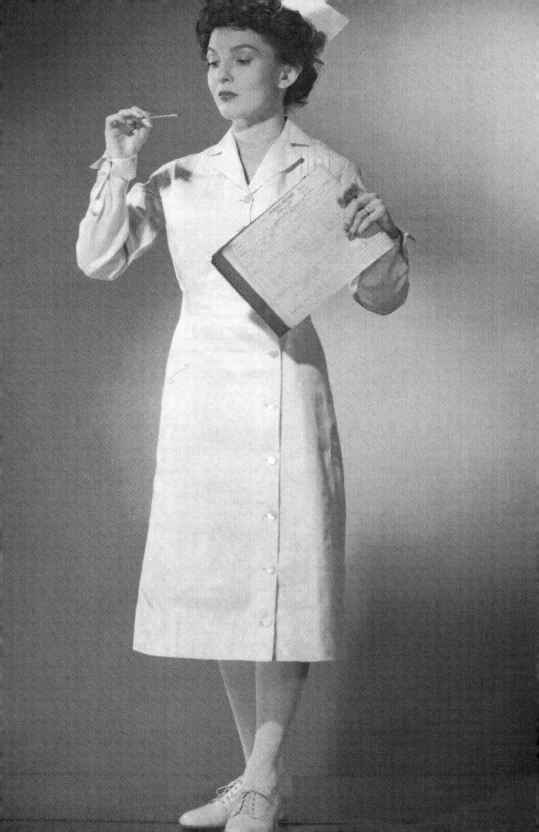

## NAUSEA

Nausea is the feeling that you are going to vomit. When your parent is on chemotherapy, one common side effect is nausea. The doctor will most likely prescribe medication to prevent nausea. But, just in case it's a good idea to have vomit bags nearby. There are designer and colorful bags you can order online.
www.morningchicnessbags.com
www.barfboutique.com

## NEIGHBORS

If you have neighbors nearby, they will probably notice changes in your parent, such as thinning hair or weight loss, that are the results of cancer treatment.

You and your parent can decide how much information you want to share with your neighbors and community. Since neighbors live so close, they could be a valuable support or help during the cancer process.

## NEW NORMAL

Cancer changes a person and changes family dynamics. Your parent's life as a cancer patient and his or her condition during and after treatment will be the new normal. A cancer diagnosis can have a profound effect on someone's life in many ways.

# NO EVIDENCE OF DISEASE (NED)

The best news you can receive is no evidence of disease. This means that the cancer does not appear on any of the tests and is pretty much gone. This is reason to celebrate!

But keep in the back of your mind that while the cancer is not large enough to show up on scans, a small tumor could still exist so don't totally let your guard down.

# NOTEBOOKS

It's a good idea to keep notebooks of your parent's doctors' appointments, symptoms and vital signs. Memories can fade and having everything written down in a central place can help you remember what your parent was like at each step of the process and how he or she has changed. If, for example, your parent has a faster heart rate than before, this may be a good thing to bring up with the doctor.

Shortly after our mom's diagnosis, we headed off to Office Max. We filled our cart with the works — binders, bright and colorful paper, dividers, and organizers — and we began to streamline the papers that had already accumulated and were beginning to be strewn around the house.

One binder was for doctor appointments. We made a section for all her visits listing the doctor she met with and the summary of the visit. We also had a section dedicated to chemotherapy — what to eat, what to expect, background on the type of chemo she was receiving and its side effects.

In the notebooks for each doctor visit, we dated each entry and always listed the type of doctor, his or her name and our questions, along with the answers. We started filling up notebooks fast so we made sure each was a different color.

If our mom wanted us to find some information about when we talked to a doctor in June, we would say, "Oh June, that was in the first notebook so that information should be in the pink notebook." Sure enough, she could find the notes she needed from that visit.

It's just as important to bring these notes and binders — or at least the recent or important ones — with you to doctors' appointments. Sometimes a doctor will ask, "What chemo are you on?" or "What amount of radiation are you given?" We were able to pull out the binder, flip to the radiation or chemotherapy section, and easily tell the doctor the answer.

It is also helpful when comparing different doctors' opinions, as one might suggest something and we can look up what another said and get a more thorough opinion given the two options.

This became especially useful when we were doctor shopping or trying to find the best surgeon to perform our mom's difficult, major and quite uncommon surgery.

## NURSES

While the doctor may prescribe the medicine or perform the surgery, the nurse is around your parent more frequently and can notice little things your parent may need.

Living in the ICU for up to seven days with our mom after surgery, we experienced the changing of the nurses and noticed how different nursing styles can really affect how the patient feels.

Some nurses were really upbeat and happy and others just did the basics of what was needed. Whatever the type of nurses your parent may have, try to communicate with them, show that you appreciate everything they are doing, and make sure you understand how they are helping your parent and how you can help the nurses help your parent.

ONCOLOGIST

OPTIMISTIC

ORGANIC

ORGANIZATIONS

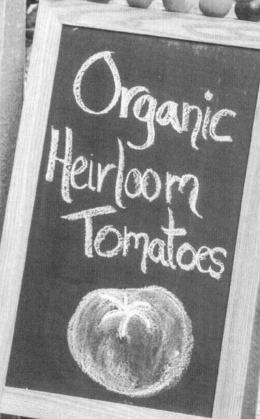

ORGANIC FARMSTAND

Organic Heirloom Tomatoes

# ONCOLOGIST

A medical doctor who specializes in the diagnosis and treatment of cancer.

# OPTIMISTIC

We tried our best to keep an optimistic attitude through this whole cancer process. It's easy to fall into doom and gloom but having an optimistic — we can beat this — attitude can go a long way in making your parent feel better and hopefully get great results.

# ORGANIC

As it relates to food, organic means that the food does not contain artificial chemicals. Organic food is becoming more popular today because many people believe that it is better to eat food that doesn't have potentially harmful chemicals.

After our mom was diagnosed, she switched to buying mostly organic foods. Organic is more expensive so if you need to be selective in what you pick to be organic, choose the foods that have a fleshier exterior. If a fruit or vegetable has a thick or tough skin — such as an avocado — it is less likely for toxins to get in versus another food with a softer more penetrable skin.

## ORGANIZATIONS

We found some non-profit organizations that focused on creating awareness of esophageal cancer, as well as supporting patients, caregivers and family members. These organizations were:

Esophageal Cancer Action Network (ECAN)
www.ecan.org

Esophageal Cancer Awareness Association (ECAA)
www.ecaware.org

There are many organizations that focus on one particularly type of cancer and help patients and family members. You can probably do a search and find one near you. They also often have local events where you can meet other people with the same type of cancer and you can get involved by volunteering or helping other people with cancer.

# P

PAIN

PARTY!

PET SCAN

PETS

PHYSICAL THERAPY (PT)

pH LEVEL

PICC LINE

POST-OP & PRE-OP

PRAYER

PROTEIN

PUBMED

PULMONARY EMBOLISM (PE)

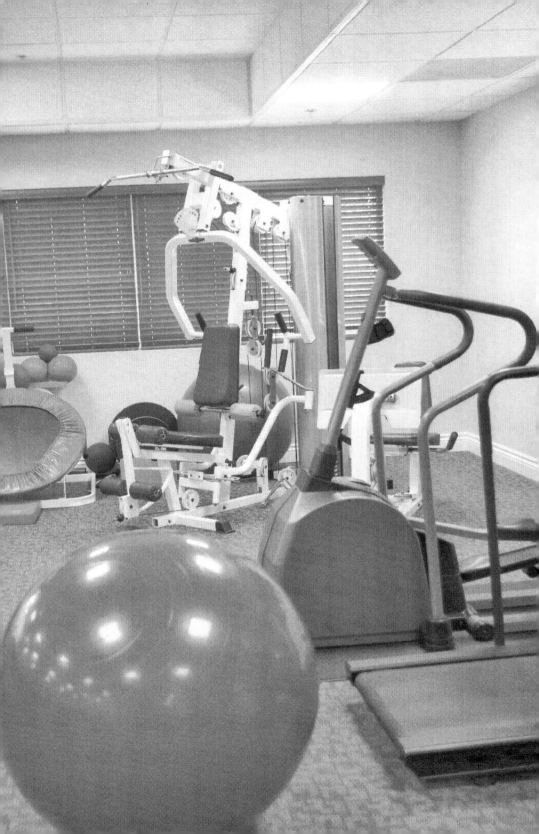

## PAIN

When you go to the doctor, your parent will be asked his or her level of pain from one to ten, one being the lowest and ten being the highest. You might want to make note of your parent's pain level to see if it is improving.

It's important to make sure your parent has effective pain medication.

## PARTY!

You're working hard to help your parent, so set aside a bit of time to party! We don't mean have a full-scale party with catering and balloons and the whole nine yards — that could be stressful. But whenever your parent reaches a milestone, like the last day of chemo or positive CT scan results, do something fun to celebrate.

Do what your family finds fun, whether that's going out to dinner, taking a walk around a lake, or going to a movie. We also had a party the night before our mom's surgery. It happened to be Jacqueline's birthday, but the party was great because it distracted us from what was to come and gave us something fun to do.

## PET SCAN

When your parent has cancer, he or she will have many tests and one might be a PET scan. PET stands for Positron Emission Tomography. It's a type of imaging that uses radioactive markers and can be used to look for signs of cancer within the body.

## PETS

When our mom was being treated with chemotherapy, the nurse gave her a calendar with the times she was most susceptible to infection because her immune system would be weakened. During those days, she was not supposed to be around our pets.

We have cats and a dog and it was very hard to keep the animals separated from her, so we had a door with glass panels installed in our hallway to separate the pets. This worked fairly well. Also, when she really wanted to see her favorite cat, she would wear gloves and a mask and just pet her for a second.

If your parent is on chemo and you have a pet that has the bad habit of drinking out of the toilet, this is a big no, no. The residual toxins from the chemo can be harmful to the pet so be sure to keep the lid down! (Also, the oncologist recommended double flushing of the toilet when our mom was being treated with chemotherapy.)

## PHYSICAL THERAPY (PT)

PT can help your parent with the mobility and function of his or her body. After our mom had surgery she couldn't stand up straight because of the three large incisions in her body that caused her to bend over, and she had very little strength in her upper body. She had physical therapy in the hospital and a physical therapist came to our home to help her regain her strength.

Our mom had three longs scars, a six-inch on her neck, seven-inch on her belly and eight-inch on her back. Some of the scars were adhering to the structure under the skin, so the physical therapist did some deep tissue massage and showed our mom how to do it so that it would heal more naturally and not be as painful.

## pH LEVEL

pH is measured on a scale of 1 to 14, with the lower numbers more acidic and the higher numbers more alkaline. Our mom tried to get her pH level higher. At the suggestion in books and from the online community, we bought pH-testing strips from Sprouts, although they are also available at other stores and online. Our mom mostly tried to increase her pH with alkaline-forming foods, but alkaline drops and other additives are also available.

## PICC LINE

PICC stands for Peripherally Inserted Central Catheter. PICC lines are an alternate way to administer the chemotherapy drug when an IV (intravenous) is not the preferred method.

A nurse or physician does the insertion of the PICC line in a hospital when the patient is awake. It takes about an hour or so. The tube, which is 25 to 60 cm in length, was inserted, in our mom's case in her arm, and up to near her heart. PICC lines can stay in place for many weeks or months but are flushed regularly at the hospital.

Our mom was on two different types of chemo drugs — Cisplatin and 5FU. They were administered through a PICC line.

If your parent has a PICC line, if it ever leaks you will probably be advised to go to the emergency room (ER). Our mom's PICC line leaked once at 3 a.m. and we went to the ER.

## POST-OP & PRE-OP

Post-op stands for postoperative. If your parent has to have surgery, the period after the surgery is called post-op. During this time, your parent starts to recover from the procedure and the anesthesia.

Pre-op stands for preoperative. It's the period before a surgical operation when your parent is getting ready to have anesthesia.

## PRAYER

We know that God has a plan but when you get the news that something horrible has happened, like your parent has cancer or a loved one has died, then you really start to question everything and just become a mess of emotions—anger, sadness and confusion.

There are different religions and beliefs, but turning toward a higher power does give a great sense of release no matter what your struggle is. We prayed that God would give us the strength to help our mom through this, through the chemo and the radiation and the surgery and the pain.

A few years ago, for our mom's birthday, we made a painting of her favorite bible verse: "This is the day the Lord hath made: we shall rejoice and be glad in it." Psalms 118:24.

We painted the verses on canvases and hung them in our home. When we asked our mom why she liked this verse, she said it reminded her to always stay positive and be happy with what God has given us. No matter what we are going through or what lies ahead, be happy, because God is with you.

When we went to church one day the pastor invited people to come to the front and be healed. We took it as a sign from God that our mom should go up and allow the pastor to dab a drop of oil onto her forehead and receive healing. God works in mysterious ways and lets Himself be known at odd times, and He definitely came through that day. The healing made us all feel a bit better, that we had some divine power on our side against this malicious enemy.

Although our mom didn't share her illness with a lot of people, the ones she did tell always offered prayer and love to her.

Many people don't know what to do when someone they know has cancer. While there is no set-in-stone code of conduct, showing the person love and offering prayer is sometimes the best and the most people can do, and it can make all the difference. A prayer both boosts a patient's spirits as well as adds one more call to God to help this person through the rough time.

## PROTEIN

Cancer patients need to make sure they eat enough protein. Your parent may feel sick from the chemotherapy and radiation and may not want to eat, but it's a good idea to encourage him or her to keep eating — especially protein.

Protein helps the body grow and repair. It can also help fight infection and strengthen the immune system. At the same time, your parent should not eat too much protein so try to find a balance. It may be a good idea to have your parent see a nutritionist to design what he or she should be eating.

This is an article on protein needs during cancer treatment:

www.oncolink.org/coping/article.cfm?c=464&id=979

Some cancer patients drink protein drinks to get the protein they need if they are not up to eating regular food. We bought many different brands but our mom could never find one that she could tolerate; however, some people she knows love them.

## PUBMED

PubMed is an online search engine that has information about scientific research and medical topics. We used PubMed to learn more about esophageal cancer. Google searches work well to find more about your parent's specific cancer, but PubMed is for scientific research articles. www.ncbi.nlm.nih.gov/pubmed

## PULMONARY EMBOLISM (PE)

When a blood clot breaks loose and travels to the lungs it is known as a pulmonary embolism or PE. If the clot is large and stops the flow of blood to the lungs, it can be deadly. About 25 percent of people with a PE die when it first happens.

Common symptoms of a PE are sudden shortness of breath, sharp chest pain from coughing or a deep breath or a cough that brings up a foamy, pink mucus.

If your parent has these symptoms it is probably a good idea to call your doctor, call 911, or go to the nearest ER.

A PE can be diagnosed by a blood test called a D-Dimer and other tests, including an ultrasound, CT scan or other tests. This link to the national heart, lung and blood institute of the National Institutes of Health lists other tests that can be done to diagnose DVT or PE.

www.nhlbi.nih.gov/health/health-topics/topics/pe/diagnosis

Our mother had a PE from a PICC line removal.

Here are some statistics about PEs and DVTs from the Center for Disease Control and Prevention:

"Estimates suggest that 60,000-100,000 Americans die [annually] of DVT/PE (also called venous thromboembolism).

- 10 to 30% of people will die within one month of diagnosis.
- Sudden death is the first symptom in about one-quarter (25%) of people who have a PE."
- www.cdc.gov/ncbddd/dvt/data.html

# QUESTIONS

# QUIET

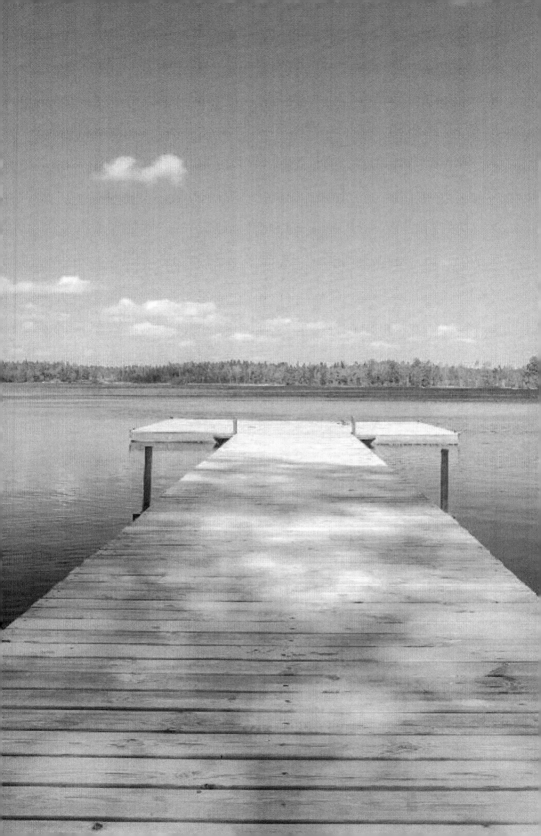

# QUESTIONS

Always make sure you have a notepad and pen or pencil with you. Write down all your questions ahead of time so that when you meet with the doctors you can ask them. At the same time, don't ask questions that you could just find answers to online, because you have limited time with the doctor.

Ask questions that pertain to your parent or that you could not find online from a trusted source.

Some people like to record the conversations with their physicians, but be sure to ask first if this is okay because not all physicians will agree to this. It's a lot faster to review notes than listen to a recorded message.

# QUIET

When your parent is undergoing cancer treatment, he or she might become hypersensitive and loud noises could be very disruptive, so it's best to talk in a quiet, calming and reassuring voice.

# R

RADIATION

RADIATION ONCOLOGIST

RECURRENCE

RESEARCH

RISKS

ROLE REVERSAL

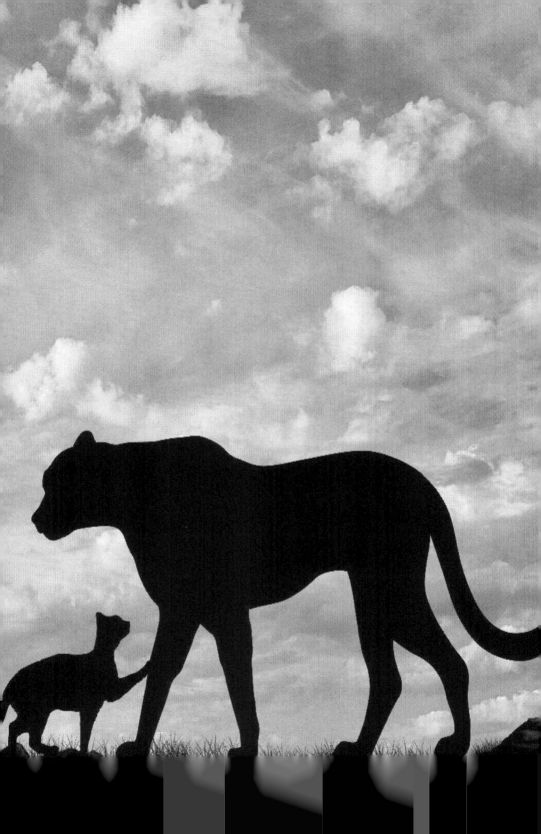

# RADIATION

Radiation is high-energy penetrating rays or subatomic particles that are used to control or treat disease. The patient lies on a table and a beam of light is aimed at the site of the tumor. The side effects of the treatment depend on where the radiation light is aimed.

The machines are very expensive and we had to drive nearly an hour each way every day for five weeks for the treatment.

The radiation won't hurt while it's happening but the cumulative effect can harm the skin or internal organs and make your parent very tired. To prevent damage to the skin, we were told to apply 100% pure aloe vera to the skin twice a day, which should be available at the pharmacy or health food store.

# RADIATION ONCOLOGIST

A radiation oncologist is a medical doctor who specializes in using radiation to treat disease. If your parent is having radiation as part of the treatment for cancer, this doctor will decide which type of treatment is best, plan the treatment, and monitor the patient.

# RECURRENCE

In the medical world, recurrence, or relapse, means the disease came back. When a patient has a recurrence it means that a test indicates cancer has returned. The recurrence can be in the same location or a different location on the body.

Recurrence is not the best word to hear, and may make you and your parent lose hope. But you should still try to keep a positive outlook. While a recurrence isn't ideal, cancer patients can keep fighting through them and good outcomes are possible with additional treatment.

## RESEARCH

In addition to the information you will get from your parent's doctors about his or her cancer, there is a ton of information on the Internet.

One good website is cancer.net.

For lots of types of cancers, it lists the following: "Overview, Statistics, Medical Illustrations, Risk Factors, Symptoms and Signs, Diagnosis, Stages, Treatment Options, About Clinical Trials, Latest Research, Coping with Side Effects, After Treatment, Questions to ask the Doctor, and Additional Resources." www.cancer.net/cancer-types

## RISKS

Risks come from dangerous situations. Life is full of risks, and surgery and cancer treatments are full of them. You and your parent should look into the possible risks and rewards of the proposed cancer treatments.

Do the risks of surgery outweigh the benefits?

For our family, we knew that the esophagectomy surgery our mom was planning to have was very risky — with a high risk of complications and with the risk of death — but we collectively decided that it was worth the risk because then hopefully the cancer would be removed and the risk of a recurrence of cancer would be smaller.

## ROLE REVERSAL

When your parent is diagnosed with cancer and undergoing treatment, if your situation is anything like ours, you will notice a sudden shift in roles. You might find that you are naturally more nurturing and independent, and you might feel the need to take on more of the responsibilities around the house.

We were very busy helping our mom organize all her treatments. In a way, we're glad we had so much to do because we were all focused on being successful and we didn't really have much time to sink into despair or reflect too much on what could happen if the treatment wasn't successful. While this might not be the approach that works for everyone, it worked for us.

# S

SCHEDULE

SCHOOL

SIDE EFFECTS

SLEEP

STAGING

STATISTICS

SUGAR

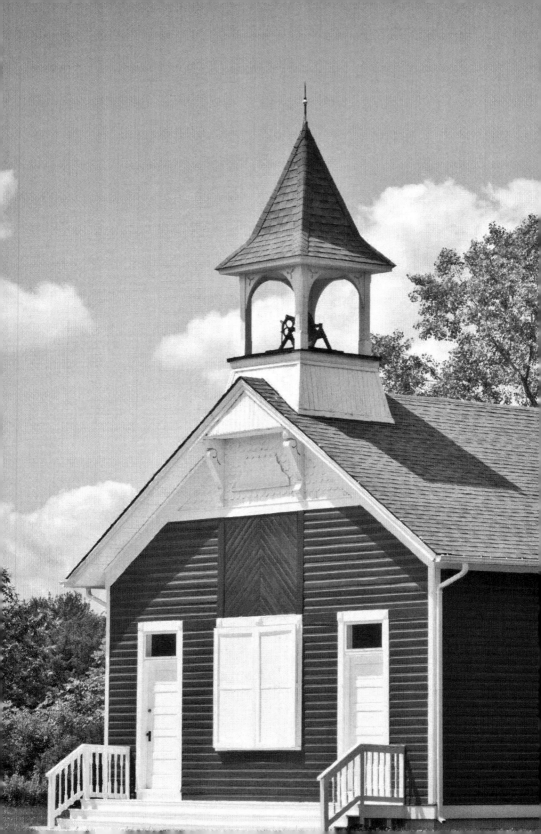

# SCHEDULE

Your parent will need a lot of help and it can be a lot of work, especially on top of homework and your other commitments. So making a schedule is a great way to stay organized and understand what you need to do. We found that a large white board with different color markers was helpful. For a while, we used an Excel spreadsheet for medications but we had trouble keeping it up to date.

# SCHOOL

Being a student is hard enough, and adding being a caregiver can be a lot to handle. It's important to be strategic with time. Try to get the most amount of schoolwork done in the least amount of time so you have enough time to both help your parent and do your work.

Make use of any time you may have. While we were waiting for the eight or so hours of our mom's esophagectomy surgery, we cracked open the books and laptops and tried to be productive with our schoolwork.

# SIDE EFFECTS

Your parent's physician will provide a list of side effects to expect from the various treatments he or she will receive. There is a huge range of side effects but cancer treatment has improved over the years and the side effects are generally not as bad as they used to be. Pretty much every side effect has a treatment and it is very important to communicate with your parent's physician when your parent gets a side effect so your parent doesn't just suffer in silence.

The side effects vary by type of cancer and type of treatment.

## SLEEP

Your parent will probably sleep a lot. Your parent will probably be very tired from all the chemotherapy drugs, radiation and doctor's appointments.

Keep this in mind and help your parent find time to rest, whether that means just lying down or taking a nap, throughout the day. You will probably also be tired from helping your parent so make sure you get enough sleep.

## STAGING

Staging is a system that classifies cancer by tumor size and how far it has spread. The lower the better. Stage 1 is better than Stage 4, but many people with Stage 4 survive, so it is always good to be optimistic. The National Cancer Institute's website has a detailed explanation of the subparts to staging.

www.cancer.gov/about-cancer/diagnosis-staging/staging

## STATISTICS

"You are not a statistic," is something people would say to us to encourage us. Even if your parent's cancer has a low survival rate — the statistics could be old and based on previous studies.

There are new treatments being developed all the time; and your parent can overcome the odds!

Statistics for specific cancers, including the chance of getting the disease and the best outcome by treatment are available on the Internet. Some people don't want to know the statistics, while others do.

Our mom looked at the statistics for different hospitals and surgeons.

It's sometimes very hard to get statistics because doctors don't have them, can't provide them or they can't easily be found on the Internet.

Scientific research studies with statistics can be found on PubMed, although they are a little difficult to understand without some medical training.

## SUGAR

In our family, we naturally have a pretty big sweet tooth. But, most sources we read said that sugar is not good for cancer patients because cancer also loves sugar.

So, our mom radically cut down on her sugar consumption. To support her efforts, we too cut down on our sugar intake. While this may or may not be hard to do depending on your desire for sugar, it's a good idea to encourage your parent to cut back on sugar and to cut back on sugar yourself too.

# T

TEACHERS

TEAM

TEARS

TENACITY

TREATMENT

TUMOR

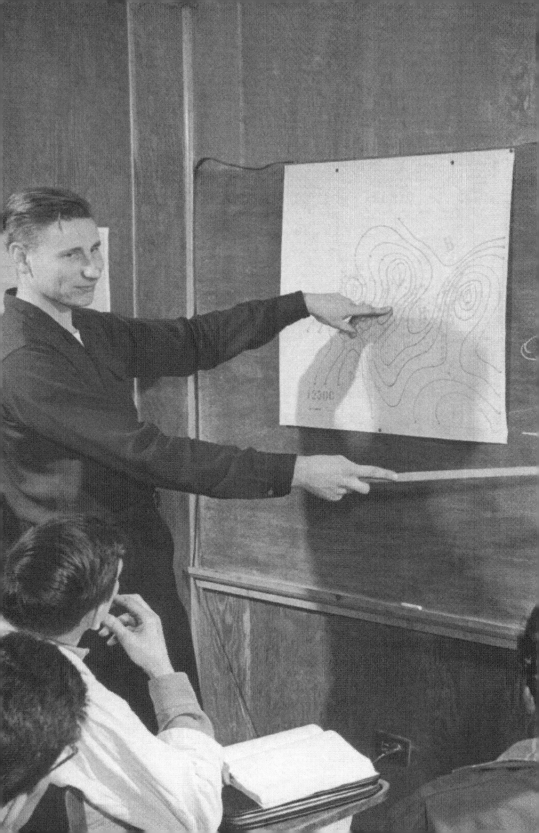

## TEACHERS

Whether you're in high school or college, you will have teachers. Depending on the size of the class, they may notice that you are acting differently because of your parent's cancer diagnosis.

Talk with your parent about whether you want to tell your teachers about your family situation. If you need to miss school to take care of your parent, especially if it's for a surgery, then it's a good idea to let your teachers know why you're missing class. They can help set you up with homework assignments so you don't miss too much of the class information.

## TEAM

After your parent's diagnosis, you should look into assembling your cancer team. Your team consists of doctors and nurses, but also your family and friends who become involved with helping your parent. We didn't tell that many family and friends, but those we did tell were very helpful. We don't know if we could have gotten through everything without them.

Some people choose to send emails to large numbers of people and organize help with food and other essentials among a large community of friends.

## TEARS

Both happy tears and sad tears can be associated with cancer. Happy when the cancer is gone or a surgery goes well and sad when there is a cancer diagnosis or bad side effects or results. We tried to keep tears — at least the sad tears — to a minimum.

Every family is different; some are very expressive and emotional, and some are more subdued. But for us it was better to keep moving forward rather than crying or reliving sad experiences.

## TENACITY

Tenacity means never giving up. Just because you have a little set back, like your parent got a complication and has to go to the emergency room, don't despair and don't give up. You will see brighter days very soon.

## TREATMENT

The major types of treatment are chemotherapy, radiation and surgery. Your parent's doctors will make recommendations and you can look up more information on the Internet to help prepare questions for the physicians.

## TUMOR

When body cells divide and grow too much, a tumor can form. Tumors can be benign or malignant. Benign is good because it means it's not cancerous; malignant means the tumor is cancerous. Tumors can appear in different parts of the body.

# U

ULTRASOUND

UNBELIEVABLE

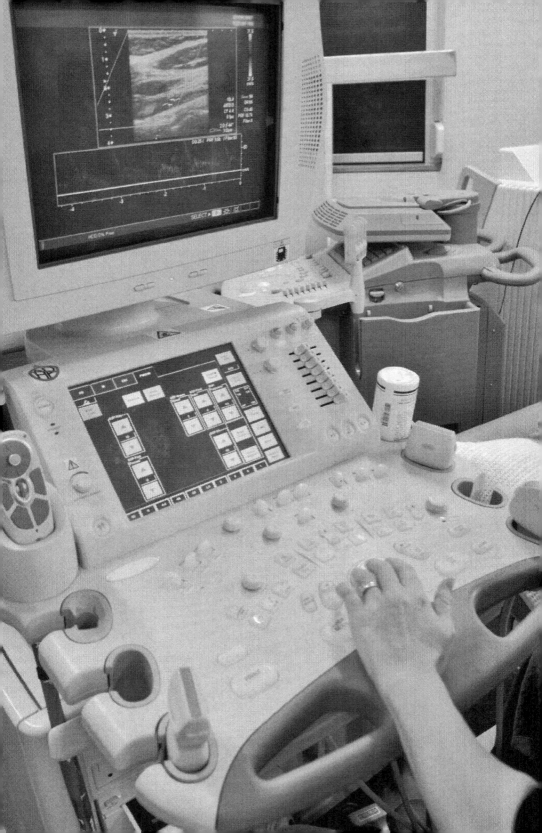

## ULTRASOUND

An ultrasound is an imaging technique that uses sound waves to visualize different parts of the body. Unlike a CT scan or a PET scan, an ultrasound cannot tell a cancerous tumor from a noncancerous one. But, using real-time images, it can tell a fluid-filled cyst from a tumor.

## UNBELIEVABLE

When your parent is diagnosed with cancer, it can seem unbelievable. You may not want to believe that it is real. The best thing to do is to accept it and do everything you can to help your parent.

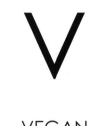

# VEGAN

# VEGETABLES

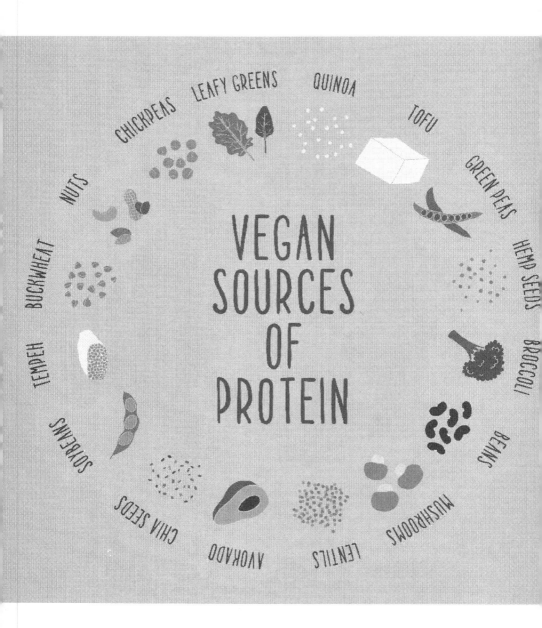

## VEGAN

A vegan is a person who doesn't eat any animal products. This includes meat as well as dairy and eggs. We read that a vegan diet was the best diet to fight cancer and after our mom was diagnosed, she chose mostly vegan foods.

## VEGETABLES

Throughout our lives, we're often told that vegetables are good for us, and they are.

We have entire books extolling the virtues of vegetables. Most books about cancer that we read strongly suggested consuming fresh organic vegetables, preferably raw, when possible.

A new book we recently found entitled, "How Not to Die: Discover the Foods Scientifically Proven to Prevent and Reverse Disease," by Michael Greger, M.D. explains in detail the benefits of a vegan diet.

# W

WAITING

WALKING

WATER-LESS SHAMPOO CAP

WHEELCHAIR

WIGS

WILLS AND TRUSTS

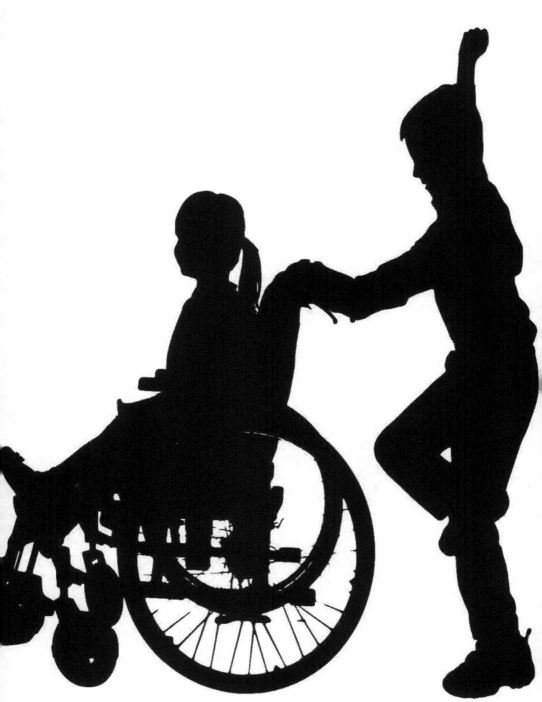

## WAITING

There is a lot of waiting involved with hospitals and diseases. You wait in the hospital waiting room, you wait at home to find out the results of a test, and you wait next to your parent in his or her hospital bed after you press the nurse call button. The best way we found to cope with waiting is just being prepared to sit for a while and bringing something to do.

## WALKING

It's good for you and your parent to stay active during the cancer process. There will be a lot of waiting and sitting, so getting up and walking in your neighborhood or on a nature walk nearby can be a great addition to the day. If your parent is recovering from surgery or a complication from treatment, he or she may have trouble walking initially so taking baby steps, literally, will help regain his or her strength.

## WATER-LESS SHAMPOO CAP

When our mom was in the hospital for 10 days she couldn't take a shower to wash her hair because she could barely stand up and she had lots of tubes connected to her. So the nurse gave us a water-less shampoo cap.

The cap, which looks like a regular shower cap, was heated for a short time in a microwave. We then put the cap on our mom's head and massaged her hair through the cap. After that, her hair was clean (although it was pretty tangled).

The water-less shampoo caps were originally developed for the NASA space program and are available online and at some pharmacies.

## WHEELCHAIRS

If your parent has trouble walking and doesn't want to stay home all the time, consider getting a wheelchair. If your insurance doesn't cover one, you can get one sent to you in a few days from places like Walmart or get a used one right away for about $20 to $50 on Craigslist.  www.craiglist.com

After our mom's pulmonary embolism, she could barely walk 50 feet, so we got a wheelchair and we could spend hours at Disneyland, at the beach or shopping.

There are two main types of wheelchairs. The type that is lighter weight and is pushed by someone is called a transport wheel-chair. The type that has large wheels that the person sitting in the chair can also operate with their hands is the other type, called a manual or standard wheelchair.

Most chairs collapse and the feet come off and they can fit in a car fairly well, but some are heavier than others.

When our mom wasn't in the wheelchair, sometimes we would play in it.

# WIGS

To respond to the changes to your parent's hair from cancer treatment, he or she may want to try a wig or hair topper, or at least buy something before the hair loss begins in order to be prepared.

A topper is like a toupee for women. It is for someone who is balding on top but still has some natural hair. It sits on top of the head and is connected with a few clips.

A few days after our mom was diagnosed, her nurse sent her a catalog from TLCDirect, which is a catalog of reasonably priced wigs, head scarves and hats. They are also available online: www.tlcdirect.org. The American Cancer Society publishes it.

While some hospital and insurance plans provide wigs and head coverings, if you are shopping for head covers TLCDirect is a good place to start, especially if you don't have time to go to a store and you want to buy a few hats, beanies, wigs or bangs just to be prepared.

The American Cancer Society also has a list of locations throughout the U.S. where cancer patients can receive a donated wig.

We Googled local wig shops and found very helpful and compassionate people who could bring us up to speed on buying a wig and who provided expertise.

The type of chemo our mom had only caused her hair to thin and she used a topper sometimes, but mostly she just wore her hair back. She didn't like the feel of a wig. Her hair is growing back thicker and curlier than before she had cancer.

## WILLS AND TRUSTS

No one wants to think about wills, but they especially don't want to think about it when it could possibly be put to use. We didn't want to have our mom redo her will because it would just make her whole illness and surgery too real. The parent might not want to think about it either. It will make it too sad for him or her, too. As the saying goes, "Plan for the worst and hope for the best." So that's what we did.

It's always a good idea to have an updated will and trust so your parent can make his or her wishes known about his or her assets. It's just a matter of making an appointment with an estate-planning lawyer, getting a list of assets, and figuring out who will be the people involved in implementing the trust and who the beneficiaries will be.

There should also be someone appointed to make medical decisions if your parent can't make them.

Be sure you know where these documents are kept.

If your parent has already started treatment, he or she might not have the energy or desire to deal with this, so you might need to encourage him or her to get this matter crossed off the list. It will be more work later if your parent hasn't done the necessary paperwork.

Our mom hadn't updated her will and trust in over 17 years so she was way overdue! Fortunately, she found an attorney who could prepare all the legal documents for her and she didn't have to drive to his office. She finally signed the papers when she got out of the hospital after her pulmonary embolism scare!

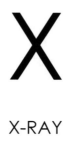

# X-RAY

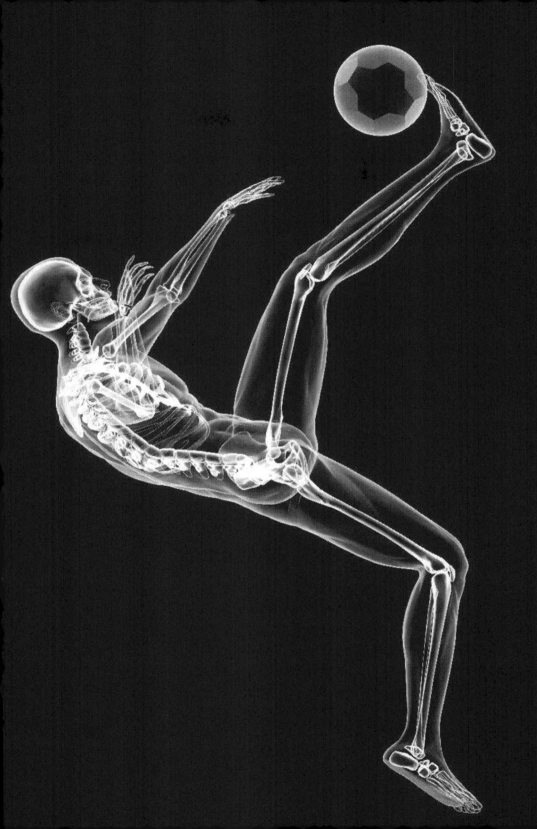

## X-RAY

If your parent needs to have his or her bones or lungs looked at, the doctor may order an x-ray. X-ray imaging looks at the inside of the body. Our mom had a lung x-ray every day when she was in the hospital after her surgery to make sure she wasn't getting pneumonia.

# Y

YOGA

YOURSELF

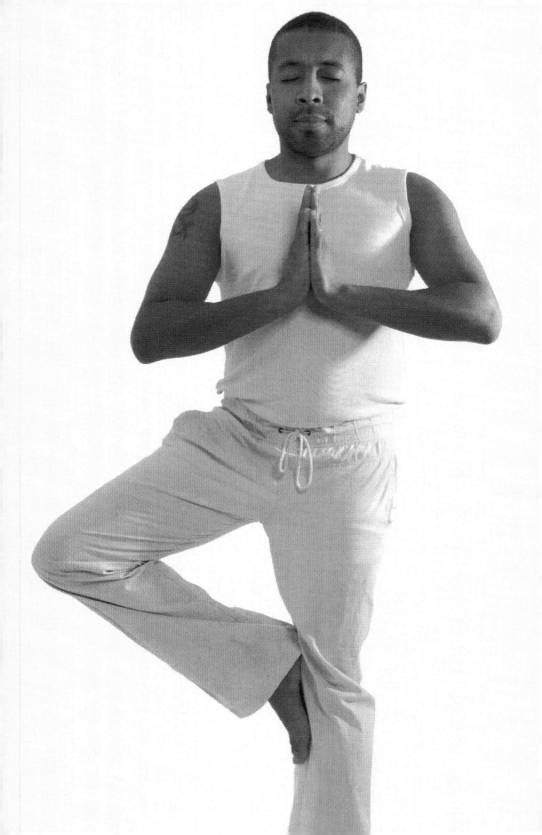

## YOGA

Yoga, like meditation, can be good for your mind and make you feel more calm and relaxed. It can also help with your flexibility and thus make your body feel better too. While you probably won't have a lot of time to go to a yoga class, you can do yoga exercises at home on a mat or on the carpet, or watch YouTube yoga videos online. It could be a fun way to bond with your parent if he or she is not feeling too sick.

## YOURSELF

In the midst of helping your parent with the cancer fight, don't forget to take care of yourself. If you're not in your best shape, then you can't help your parent as well. Make sure you're eating right and getting enough sleep and try to delegate work among your team that you and your parent assembled. It shouldn't all fall on you.

# Z

ZOBOOMAFOO

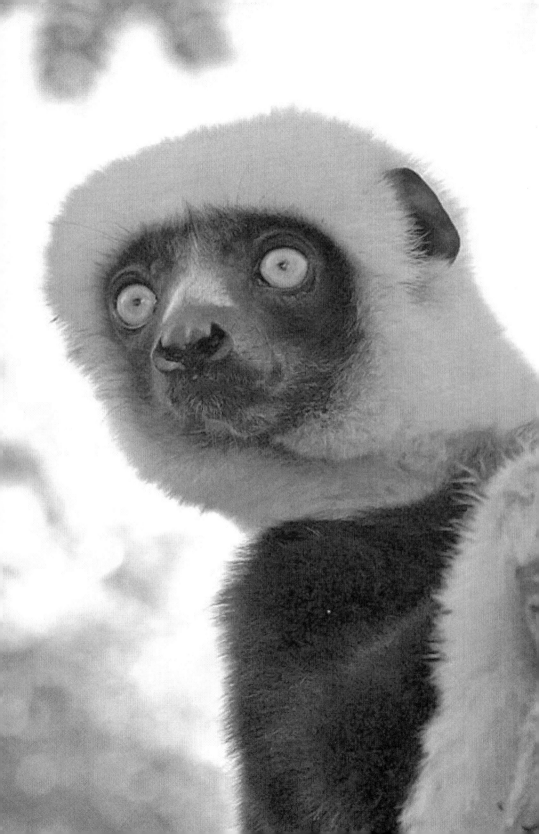

# ZOBOOMAFOO

The first preschool wildlife show on PBS about animals, popular in the 1990s was called Zoboomafoo. We grew up watching Zoboomafoo and the Kratt brothers jumping around and playing with lemurs and new animals on every episode.

This show, along with Crocodile Hunter, helped instill in us a love for animals and, looking back, helped develop our nurturing spirit.

We think taking care of animals helped us to become responsible and able to help our mom as much as we did. Our mom pretty much let us have any pet we wanted, but we had to take care of it ourselves.

Before we took care of our mom, we cared for rabbits, cats and dogs at home. We had miniature donkeys at a stable. We also talked our mom into letting us get chickens, ducks, fish, frogs, birds, and turtles and we rescued a crayfish that we found on the street.

# ABOUT THE AUTHORS

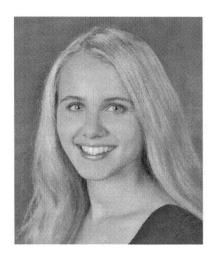

*Katherine Carr*

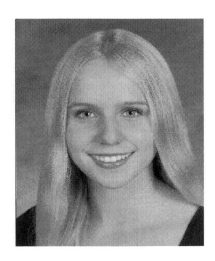

*Jacqueline Carr*

KATHERINE CARR and JACQUELINE CARR are sisters who share an interest in scientific research and writing. They both put their lives on hold to help their mother after her diagnosis with a rare and deadly cancer.

Both Katherine and Jacqueline have performed cancer research at the University of California, Irvine, and stem cell research at Stanford University. Additionally, they have both written articles for *The Stanford Daily* and the *Orange County Register*.

Katherine is currently a junior at Stanford University majoring in chemistry, with a minor in communications, while Jacqueline is a senior in high school in Irvine, California. Their mother shows no signs of the disease two years after treatment.

Made in the USA
San Bernardino, CA
02 March 2016